The Prediabetes
Action Plan and Cookbook

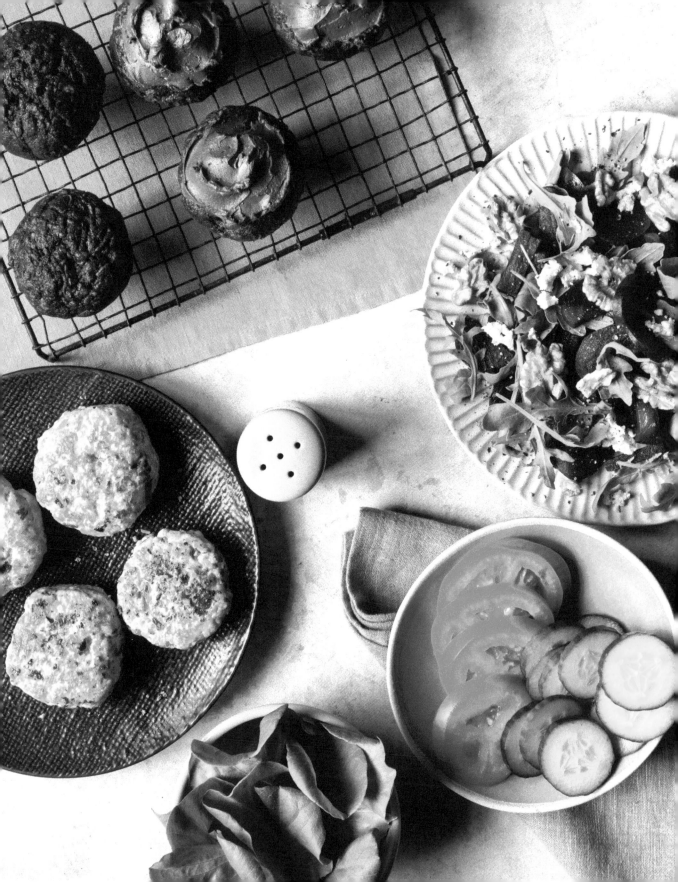

THE
Prediabetes
Action Plan
— AND COOKBOOK —

A Simple Guide to Getting Healthy and Reversing Prediabetes

CHERYL MUSSATTO, MS, RD, LD

PHOTOGRAPHY BY NADINE GREEFF

ROCKRIDGE
PRESS

Interior and Cover Designer: Joshua Moore
Art Producer: Sara Feinstein
Editor: Bridget Fitzgerald
Production Editor: Andrew Yackira
Photography: © 2019 Nadine Greeff
Author photo courtesy of © Tommy Peterson of T. H. Peterson Photography
Cover Recipe: Greek-Style Turkey Burgers, page 88

ISBN: Print 978-1-64152-474-2
eBook 978-1-64152-475-9

To the millions of people living with prediabetes; you're an inspiration in your quest to make your health a priority.

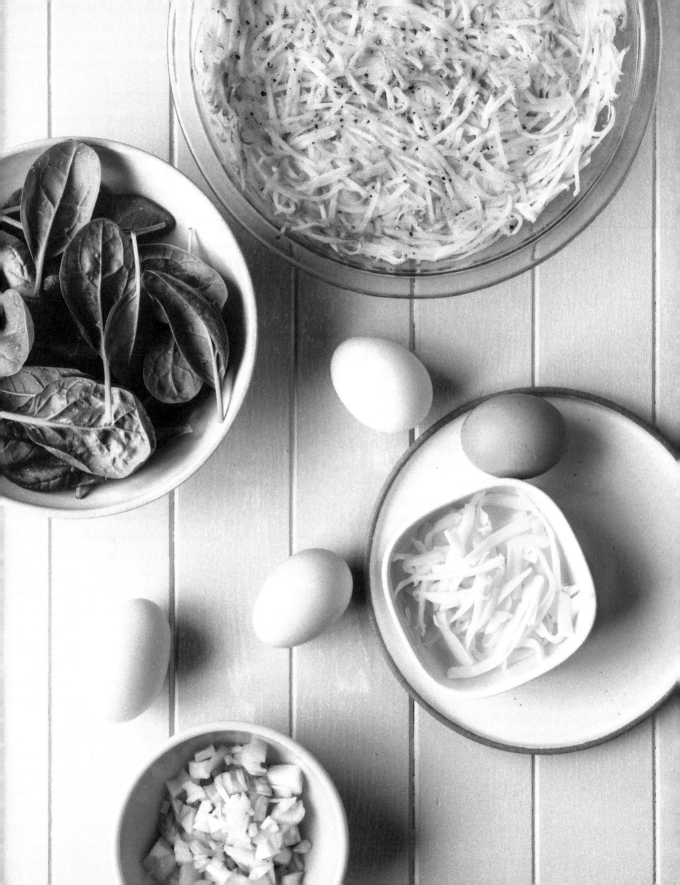

Contents

Introduction

Chances are you're holding this book because you've been diagnosed with prediabetes. It's not something anyone wants to hear. You're probably thinking, "I don't have time for this," or, "Why me?" That's perfectly normal. No one anticipates developing a health condition—and all of us would prefer not to deal with one.

While a diagnosis of prediabetes can be disheartening, let's look at it from another viewpoint. Prediabetes is not the same as type 2 diabetes. Yes, it can lead to type 2 diabetes, but it doesn't have to. You see, you've been given a gift: Your elevated blood sugar was discovered early. If months or years had elapsed, you'd likely be facing a diagnosis of type 2 diabetes—without having had the chance to forestall it. You've been given a glimpse into your future health with time to spare to make the necessary lifestyle and dietary changes. What an opportunity!

As a registered dietitian, I have had the privilege of helping people live their healthiest lives. My career as a health care professional spans more than 30 years, and I've worn many hats over that time. From working in county health departments, doctors' offices, and long-term-care facilities to my roles as an adjunct professor in a community college, a freelance health/nutrition writer, and a director of the dietary department in a hospital, I've enjoyed a variety of experiences as a dietitian. But my experience as a clinical dietitian in an endocrinology clinic has been the most challenging and rewarding. Every day I see clients who want and deserve answers to living their healthiest lives—and I get to help them figure out the intricacies of eating, exercise, and living their best lives ever. When patients meet their health goals, I get to share in the celebration of their achievements.

That's what inspired this book—my desire to put you on the path toward achieving overall wellness while beating back prediabetes. Think of it as your blueprint for developing a new and better relationship with food, with me to guide you every step of the way. No need to feel overwhelmed or worried—and you won't have to give up all your favorite foods, either.

This book takes the guesswork out of what to eat and how to get physically active. You can expect the following:

» A 2-week starter meal and activity plan (see page 33) that will get you on the right track toward cooking nutritious meals and practicing healthy habits

» 75 easy and delicious recipes that offer a wide array of healthy foods you can feel good about enjoying

» An explanation of how nutrients in food affect your blood sugar so you can make informed decisions when it comes to your diet and lifestyle

» Guidelines for increasing physical activity, getting adequate sleep, and setting goals to establish new health habits to aid you in reversing prediabetes

Remember, you are in charge of your health. This book is your action plan so you can reverse prediabetes in a manageable way with the goal of preventing diabetes. Before you know it, you'll be living a healthier lifestyle without prediabetes. Let's get started!

TAKING
ACTION

Action. Embrace this word. You'll soon see how easy it is to take action when your goal is to defeat prediabetes and reclaim your health. Every day, opportunities will present themselves. Seize those moments. Neglecting your body's needs will only hurt you in the long run—inactivity is like giving up. There's no need for a defeatist attitude when taking action can start with a few small, achievable steps that anyone can manage. And it could mean the difference between enjoying a long, healthy life or facing a future diagnosis of type 2 diabetes and all the complications that accompany it.

The first step is learning what prediabetes is and the role of nutrition in treating it. Then I'll show you how to stock your kitchen with the right foods for success, and how to get started with the 2-week meal plan. It's everything you need to set you on a path toward a lifetime of health and wellness.

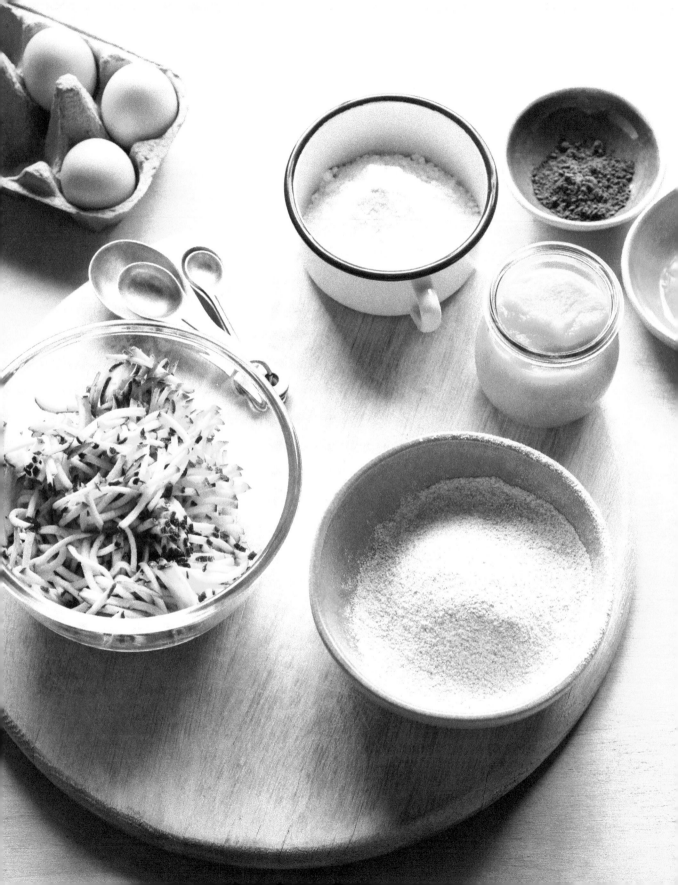

ONE

Understanding Prediabetes

The numbers keep rising, and they're hard to ignore. Not that long ago, it was estimated that 79 million adults in the United States had prediabetes. Today, that number has grown to 84 million. Even more alarming is that out of that number, only 12 percent have been diagnosed. That means over 70 million individuals are unknowingly walking around with prediabetes and are at increased risk of developing type 2 diabetes, one of the leading causes of morbidity and mortality.

Prediabetes is a strong risk factor for developing type 2 diabetes. The good news is that a diagnosis of prediabetes does not automatically mean you will develop type 2 diabetes. Instead it is a wake-up call that, metabolically, things have gone awry. Your blood glucose level is higher than normal, but below the level of diabetes. Luckily, you have been diagnosed at an early stage of the disease, allowing you time to potentially reverse it. Lifestyle changes are required, but they do not have to be disruptive. The good habits of diet and exercise that can reverse prediabetes are the same good habits that everyone, whether or not they have prediabetes, should practice for a healthy and happy life. Be proactive—you have already taken the first step. When you take action to manage prediabetes, the odds are in your favor.

Diabetes and Prediabetes

A diagnosis of prediabetes, or even diabetes, can come as a complete surprise. Symptoms are often vague or nonexistent. Yet prediabetes and diabetes have become two of the biggest epidemics of the twenty-first century. Likely, you have friends or family members who have been diagnosed.

In the United States, both prediabetes and type 2 diabetes have become increasingly prevalent in recent years, due in part to the standard American diet. Americans tend to eat larger portion sizes, especially at restaurants, where people increasingly get their meals; they also consume greater quantities of sugary beverages and eat fewer fresh fruits and vegetables. Additionally, the rise of "fat-free" foods, which replace fat with sugar, and more stressful lifestyles can lead to emotional eating—eating for comfort rather than due to hunger. All these factors have contributed to the rise of obesity in the United States over the past 30 years, which also correlates with the rise in both prediabetes and type 2 diabetes.

THE DIFFERENCE

The terms *prediabetes* and *diabetes* can be confusing. Health care professionals use different parameters and blood glucose tests to diagnose and distinguish between the two. If you have an abnormal result, you will likely have a second test to confirm your diagnosis.

What is prediabetes? A prediabetes diagnosis simply means your blood glucose levels are higher than normal, but not high enough to be classified as full-blown diabetes. You may hear the term "borderline diabetes" and wonder if this is the same thing as prediabetes. Rarely used anymore, the term can create confusion depending on how some people define it. Some use it to define prediabetes while others define it as type 2 diabetes managed without medications. Ask for clarification if a health care professional uses this term.

What is diabetes? Diabetes is a chronic and progressive disease that occurs when the body doesn't produce enough insulin, leading to an excess of sugar, or glucose, in the blood. Insulin, a hormone produced by your pancreas, helps your body use the glucose found in foods containing carbohydrates as fuel, or energy. Glucose is required by all your body's cells to function properly.

When sufficient insulin is unavailable or impaired, your cells are unable to use the glucose as fuel and it builds up in the bloodstream, reaching elevated levels. Your body will try to compensate by excreting excess glucose in your urine.

To get a greater sense of the magnitude of prediabetes and diabetes, the latest statistics from the *National Diabetes Statistics Report, 2017,* from the Centers for Disease Control and Prevention, reveal the number of Americans affected by diabetes is growing.

» Slightly more than 9 percent of the population, 30 million American adults, had diabetes in 2015.

» Of those 30 million adults, 76 percent, or about 23 million, were diagnosed, and the remaining 24 percent, about 7 million, were undiagnosed.

» Every year an additional 1.5 million Americans are newly diagnosed with diabetes.

» As of 2015, diabetes remained the seventh leading cause of death in the United States.

» In the United States alone, the total cost of diagnosed diabetes in 2017, including direct medical care and lost productivity, such as absenteeism, was $327 billion.

Diabetes affects all races and ethnicities. Consider the following, for people ages 20 and older diagnosed with diabetes:

» 7.4 percent of non-Hispanic whites

» 8 percent of Asian-Americans

» 12.1 percent of Hispanics

» 12.7 percent of African-Americans (of non-Hispanic origin)

» 15.1 percent of American Indians / Alaska Natives

More recent data collected from the Gallup-Sharecare Well-Being Index found the rate of diabetes increased in 18 states in the United States over the past decade, with no states showing a decrease. This is why it is so important to prevent diabetes while you have the chance.

TYPE 1 AND TYPE 2

The two types of diabetes are called type 1 diabetes and type 2 diabetes. Understanding the differences between them is important for understanding how to prevent prediabetes from turning into type 2.

	TYPE 1	TYPE 2
PERCENTAGE OF CASES	5 to 10 percent	90 to 95 percent
AGE OF ONSET	Most often develops in individuals under 21, but can occur at any age	Typically diagnosed in individuals over 40, but can occur at younger ages, even in children
CAUSE OF ONSET	Destruction of pancreatic beta cells resulting in little, if any, insulin made; considered an autoimmune disease	Pancreas producing insufficient insulin or due to insulin resistance
RISK FACTORS	Viral infections, family history Note: Prediabetes is NOT a risk factor for type 1 diabetes.	Older age, family history of diabetes, obesity, prior history of gestational diabetes, physical inactivity, certain races or ethnicities, prediabetes
REQUIRES INSULIN	Always	Sometimes
OLDER NAMES KNOWN BY	Juvenile-onset diabetes, insulin-dependent diabetes mellitus	Adult-onset diabetes, non-insulin-dependent diabetes mellitus
TREATMENT	Insulin therapy, multiple daily self-monitoring glucose testing, oral medications, regular exercise, and a healthy diet	Controlled-carbohydrate healthy meal plan, weight loss if necessary, regular exercise, self-monitoring glucose testing, oral medications, and possibly insulin at some point

INSULIN RESISTANCE

Insulin resistance is the hallmark of both prediabetes and type 2 diabetes. To get a better understanding, let's break it down.

Our bodies require glucose, a necessary source of energy for the body's cells. When we eat foods containing carbohydrates, the carbohydrates are broken down into a sugar called glucose. When glucose enters the bloodstream, the pancreas (a large gland sitting behind the stomach) detects a rise in blood glucose levels and secretes the hormone insulin into the bloodstream. Insulin's job is to help move the glucose from the bloodstream into the body's cells, providing energy, or to store it for later use.

When a person is insulin resistant, the pancreas still produces insulin in response to increased blood glucose levels, but cells in your muscles, fat, and liver do not allow sufficient glucose to enter. This weak response by the cells leads to elevated blood glucose levels. The pancreas then has to make more insulin, and, over time, the pancreas may wear out. Most people with insulin resistance are unaware they have it, but eventually, the worn-out pancreas no longer produces enough insulin to overcome the cells' resistance, resulting in higher blood glucose levels (prediabetes) and, ultimately, type 2 diabetes.

RISK FACTORS AND SYMPTOMS

The risk factors for prediabetes are basically the same as for type 2 diabetes (see chart on page 6) and include the following:

» Being age 45 or older
» Being of African American, Hispanic and Latino, American Indian, Asian American, or Pacific Islander ethnicity
» Being overweight or obese

» Family history of diabetes
» Having polycystic ovary syndrome (PCOS)
» History of gestational diabetes
» History of heart disease or stroke
» Physical inactivity

The condition of prediabetes is sneaky; it has no symptoms, which is why the majority of people who currently have prediabetes don't know it. Routine blood tests often lead to diagnosis. However, some people with prediabetes may develop what's called acanthosis nigricans, characterized by velvety dark patches appearing in body folds such as the neck, armpits, elbows, hands, groin, and knees.

How to Reverse Prediabetes

If the US rates of diabetes will ever begin a downward trend, the focus must be on prevention. Your diagnosis is part of that effort: Guidelines for blood sugar levels that qualify as prediabetes have been developed as a proactive approach. Lifestyle interventions, such as increasing physical activity, are the primary method of normalizing blood glucose levels and reversing prediabetes. Earlier and more frequent detection can lead to better chances, and remember that reversing the condition requires accountability to yourself and to your health. As with all change, it may take some time and commitment, but it is completely doable.

A question you may have is: *Can diabetes be cured?* The short answer is, it depends on when you are diagnosed. Being diagnosed at a prediabetic stage is promising, but most people with type 2 diabetes likely have had the disease for several years. They can't turn back the clock, but they can adopt healthy lifestyle habits to manage their diabetes, keep their bodies healthy, and reduce serious complications.

That's why a prediabetes diagnosis gives you a greater chance of dodging diabetes. Don't despair—be hopeful: Now is the time to take action.

A Healthy Diet

The biggest influence on your success isn't a *diet* in the trendy, fad-diet sense but a healthy way of eating. Regardless of whether a person has a diagnosis of prediabetes, everyone should have a basic knowledge of the fundamentals of human nutrition.

Understanding how food nourishes the human body and which foods best serve your health will help you make appropriate food choices, plan healthy meals, and design a diet to support your goals. Learning about key nutrients in foods and using the dietary guidelines to apply this knowledge puts you in control of what goes on your plate—and into your body.

NUTRIENTS

You may not feel like it, but you have been given a second chance—and the best place to begin is by taking an in-depth look at your current eating habits. Having prediabetes does not mean you have to follow any specific "diet." In fact, the word "diet" simply means "way of eating." Everyone eats, so each of us is on a "diet." Think of your diet as your eating plan to good health. You require the same nutrients as someone without prediabetes.

WHAT NOW? QUESTIONS TO ASK YOUR DOCTOR

After your diagnosis, you'll have many questions. Here are five worth asking your doctor:

1

What is causing my high blood sugar?
This million-dollar question will help you better understand the underlying risk factors for prediabetes.

2

What goals should I set to lower my blood sugar?
Realistic goal setting is crucial. Goals should address your target blood glucose range, weight, exercise, dietary changes, and lifestyle modifications.

3

Can I be referred to a registered dietitian?
Food choices have the biggest impact on your blood glucose levels, so it's critical to eat a balanced diet (and eat meals at consistent times) to help manage blood glucose levels. A registered dietitian can create a customized eating plan tailored to your age, medical needs, fitness level, lifestyle, and food preferences.

4

What kind of exercise is important?
Regular exercise not only improves your overall health but also reduces your risk for diabetes. Physical activity creates a demand for energy, thereby using excess glucose and improving how insulin works. Consult your doctor for appropriate ways to increase your physical activity.

5

Are there specialists I should see?
Elevated blood glucose levels can lead to various complications—all over the body—as over time, they damage your blood vessels (both large and small). This damage can lead to everything from nervous system problems to blindness, which is why type 2 diabetes is so serious. By controlling your blood glucose, blood pressure, and cholesterol according to your treatment plan, you can help reduce your risk. Schedule yearly appointments with an optometrist or ophthalmologist for a comprehensive eye exam to detect any retina or vision changes, and with a podiatrist for a foot exam to prevent ulcers and other complications.

Nutrition is a fascinating topic. Every day our bodies renew their structures by continuously building a little muscle, skin, and bone and replacing old tissues with new. The building blocks that accomplish this amazing feat come from the foods we eat, and the best foods provide proper nutrients to support this growth and maintenance of strong muscles and bones, healthy skin, and sufficient blood to cleanse and nourish your body. That means it's really important to eat foods that provide the proper amount of calories for energy, as well as nutrients such as water, carbohydrates, protein, fat, vitamins, and minerals.

A well-chosen diet supplying the right combination of each nutrient can have a profoundly positive effect.

Carbohydrates

Carbohydrates, as your body's main source of energy, are the ideal nutrient to meet its energy needs. Providing four calories of energy per gram, carbohydrates supply fuel to your cells and brain, primarily in the form of glucose, the predominate sugar in carbohydrate foods.

Quality carbohydrates, found naturally in all plant-based foods such as whole grains, fruits, vegetables, nuts, and legumes (dried beans and peas), are healthier as they're loaded with a variety of vitamins, minerals, fiber, antioxidants, and phyto-chemicals that keep your body functioning at its best. And because plants do not use all the stored glucose they make, extra glucose is available for us to use when we consume those foods. The only animal-based foods containing carbohydrates are milk, yogurt, and cottage cheese. Other animal-based foods—beef, poultry, pork, lamb, fish, butter, eggs, or cheese—do not contain carbohydrates.

Not-as-nutritious *refined carbohydrates* from highly processed foods, such as sugary beverages, candy, desserts, and snack foods like pretzels and chips, have had most of their nutrients and fiber removed and are higher in sugar and/or fat. For this reason, they are often considered "empty" calories—calories, but with few nutrients that benefit the body.

All foods containing carbohydrates are eventually broken down by your body into glucose. Glucose is absorbed through the walls of your small intestine into your bloodstream and is then known as blood glucose or blood sugar. When your pancreas detects rising blood glucose, it releases insulin to clear the excess sugar out of your blood, moving it into cells for energy. But for those with insulin resistance, the body's cells don't respond to insulin's efforts to unlock their doors. The pancreas then secretes more insulin into the blood, but with minimal effect. Excess circulating glucose—unused energy—can lead to feelings of fatigue and hunger, which, in turn, can make you hungrier for more refined or sugary carbohydrate foods—a common way we tend to curb hunger.

WHAT IS STARCH?

Starch is a type of carbohydrate, also referred to as a complex carbohydrate because it is made up of long chains of sugar molecules. Healthy starchy foods include peas, corn, potatoes, pasta, beans, rice, and grains. Starches are a more concentrated source of carbohydrates and calories than, say, fruits or nonstarchy vegetables (such as broccoli, tomatoes, asparagus, and cauliflower), but many of them are excellent sources of fiber, vitamins, minerals, and phytochemicals. They are an important part of a healthy, well-balanced diet when consumed in reasonable portions.

In time this becomes a vicious cycle of eat, feel tired and hungry, eat some more. The pancreas continues to pump out insulin in response to increased blood sugar levels, but the resistant cells disregard the insulin, and the excess glucose gets stored as fat, leading to weight gain—and you still feel tired and hungry, so you eat again....

Even those with prediabetes need to eat carbohydrates every day, but the more you eat, the higher your blood glucose may rise. Keep portion sizes reasonable (see page 16, Building a Healthy Plate), and choose carbohydrate-containing foods providing plenty of vitamins, minerals, and fiber, and eat less of those high in sugar or refined grains such as white flour.

Protein

Protein is an amazing and versatile nutrient. Recognized more than 150 years ago as being vital for life, the word "protein" comes from the Greek word *proteios*, meaning "of prime importance."

Proteins perform many vital functions in your body including gene regulation, the production of digestive enzymes, hormones, and antibodies, and strengthening bones, teeth, skin, tendons, cartilage, blood vessels, and other tissues. Essentially, protein is an integral component to the workings of a healthy body.

Like carbohydrates, proteins also provide four calories of energy per gram and are found in a variety of both animal- and plant-based foods. When choosing the best protein sources, it's good to include foods high in protein but low in fat. Some plant-based proteins include beans, lentils, split peas, edamame, tempeh, tofu, hummus, and spreads such as almond butter, cashew butter, or peanut butter. They vary in how much fat and carbohydrates they contain, so read the labels.

Animal sources of protein include fatty fish, such as salmon, tuna, and mackerel; poultry without the skin; lean beef and pork; eggs; and dairy products. Since most animal sources of protein do not contain carbohydrates (with the exception of milk, yogurt, and cottage cheese), they do not raise blood glucose levels.

A balanced meal plan usually has 3 to 5 ounces of meat or a plant protein source at each meal. Proteins take longer to digest, which also slows the digestion of carbohydrates, resulting in a slower rate of glucose entering your bloodstream.

Fats

Get ready for a surprise—you won't find a "fats are bad for you" lecture here. Actually, fats are a valuable and necessary nutrient. It all boils down to two factors—quality and quantity.

Just like carbohydrates and protein, fats provide calories but contain more than twice the amount per gram, at nine calories each; so, eating a high-fat diet can of course result in weight gain.

But fat has many jobs for keeping us healthy. Fat forms the major material of cell membranes, is the body's main form of stored energy, helps our body absorb vitamins, and enhances our enjoyment of eating. Fats are divided into those that are healthy and unhealthy.

Healthy fats include polyunsaturated, monounsaturated, and omega-3 fatty acids, all playing a role in reducing heart disease. The best food sources of poly- and monounsaturated healthy fats include vegetable oils such as olive, canola, flaxseed, grapeseed, and walnut; avocados; olives; nuts such as almonds, pecans, pistachios, and walnuts; and seeds such as flax, pumpkin, chia, and sesame. Be sure to include heart-healthy omega-3 fatty acids when planning meals. They include albacore tuna, mackerel, halibut, herring, salmon, sardines, and trout.

Unhealthy fats are saturated and trans fats. These "bad fats" can clog arteries, increasing your risk of heart disease. Foods containing a large amount of saturated fats include coconut and palm oils, lard, shortening, butter, cream cheese, sour cream, margarine, bacon, cream, and high-fat meats such as ground chuck or prime rib. In recent years, the U.S. Food and Drug Administration (FDA) has slowly banned trans fats in processed foods, resulting in a majority of food manufacturers cutting back on trans fat use. However, trans fats may still be in some foods such as crackers, cookies, cakes, frozen pies, and other baked goods. Read nutrition labels, and choose foods with 0 grams of trans fats. Avoid foods that contain "partially hydrogenated oil" in the ingredient list, as those can contain up to 0.49 grams of trans fats and still list 0 grams on the label.

Like protein, fats do not contain sugar and, therefore, have little effect on your blood glucose. Even though unsaturated fats have many health aspects, be aware of the quantities you consume. A goal of no more than 30 percent of calories from fat, mostly plant-based unsaturated fats, is a reasonable and safe one for anyone with prediabetes or insulin resistance.

Besides controlling blood glucose levels and carbohydrate intake, you should also pay attention to other nutrients such as fiber and sodium. Remember, it's the diet as a whole that contributes to overall health, weight management, and blood sugar control.

Fiber is the indigestible part of plant foods (fiber is only found in plant-based foods; no animal foods contain it), and it is lacking in most American diets. The *Dietary Guidelines for Americans* states that the adequate intake (AI) for dietary fiber is 25 grams per day for women and 38 grams per day for men. Because fiber takes longer to process in the body, it keeps you feeling fuller longer and, therefore, helps reduce the chances you'll overeat. Examples of high-fiber foods include beans, lentils, and legumes; fruits and vegetables, especially with an edible skin; nuts and seeds; whole grains such as quinoa or barley; and whole-grain breads, pastas, and some cereals.

Sodium is a mineral that does have important functions, but it is still wise to be mindful and reduce your intake to keep blood pressure low (prediabetes may increase your risk of developing high blood pressure, a leading cause of heart disease and stroke). How much sodium you require depends on several factors— age, history of high blood pressure, and ethnicity. But you can safely follow the advice of three well-respected health groups: the American Diabetes Association, the American Heart Association, and the *2015–2020 Dietary Guidelines for Americans*. Each states that limiting sodium intake to no more than 2,300 milligrams (mg) per day and no less than 1,500 mg per day is a safe bet.

Be aware that sodium amounts add up quickly. In a typical day of eating, you might have a bowl of cereal with milk for breakfast (250 mg sodium), a cup of canned soup with a turkey sandwich for lunch (2,200 mg sodium), and a slice of pizza and salad with light dressing for dinner (710 mg sodium). Add these meals together, and the total sodium for one day equals 3,160 mg—well above the recommended intake. Other high-sodium foods include processed tomato products and salad dressings; snack foods such as chips, crackers, and pretzels; and frozen meals.

To lower your sodium intake, try the following: Eat more fresh fruit, vegetables, and low-fat dairy; season foods with lemon juice or salt-free herb blends instead of salt; limit processed meats; taste food first before adding additional salt; and read nutrition labels. Low-sodium foods have less than 140 mg per serving.

HEART-HEALTHY FOODS

Heart health is another goal to focus on. Heart disease is the leading cause of illness and death in people with type 2 diabetes. The connection between diabetes and heart disease starts with high blood glucose levels. Over time, high glucose in the bloodstream can damage the arteries, causing them to become stiff and hard. Fatty material builds up on the inside of these blood vessels and creates a condition called atherosclerosis, which can eventually block blood flow to the heart or brain. A person's risk of heart disease with diabetes is further increased if they also have a family history of cardiovascular disease or stroke. Start good habits now to include more heart-healthy foods. Here are some dos and don'ts:

» Aim for 2 to 3 servings of fatty fish, such as salmon, tuna, mackerel, herring, or sardines, each week.

» Eat at least 5 servings of fruits and vegetables daily.

» Include heart-healthy fats such as olive, canola, or avocado oils; nuts and nut butters; seeds; and avocado in your dishes.

» Include whole grains, such as oatmeal, barley, quinoa, buckwheat, or farro, in your meals.

» Do not consume more than 2,300 mg of sodium each day.

» Avoid high–saturated fat and sodium-rich processed meats, such as salami, hot dogs, sausage, bacon, and bologna.

» Avoid highly refined and processed grains, such as white bread, white rice, and low-fiber breakfast cereals.

» Limit your intake of added sugars found in sweetened beverages and other processed foods.

COMMON HIDDEN-SUGAR FOODS

As you've already learned, most foods contain carbohydrates, which break down into the sugar glucose and affect your blood sugar levels. Some carbohydrates digest slowly, while others digest quickly. *Slow-digesting carbs* cause your blood sugar to rise at a consistent rate, like a slow trickle of sugar entering your bloodstream. *Fast-digesting carbs* cause your blood sugar to spike quickly with a flood of glucose that is difficult for your body to process.

Some of the following fast-digesting foods may surprise you:

» White rice

» Any foods made with refined white flours (breads, pastas, cereals)

» Any foods with added sugars (muffins, cakes, cookies, all sugary beverages, fruit juice)

» Potato chips, pretzels, and crackers

1. Serving Size: Look here first. All the information on the label is based on the serving size of the food. This example shows that the package contains 8 servings, but the serving size information provided is for only 1 serving. So, if you had a two-serving portion, all numbers listed would be doubled.

2. Calories: If your goal is losing weight, look at the calories per serving. Choose products that are lower in calories per serving.

3. % Daily Value (DV):
This is based on nutrient recommendations for a 2,000-calorie diet, but you may need more or less per day. This percentage allows you to compare and evaluate foods with regard to nutrient and calorie contents and how that food fits into your daily meal plan.

A DV of 5 percent or less is considered low. Aim low in saturated fat, trans fat, cholesterol, and sodium.

A DV of 20 percent or more is considered high, or a good source of that nutrient. Aim high in vitamins, minerals, and fiber.

4. Saturated Fat and Trans Fat: Reducing these fats helps cut your risk of heart disease, so choose products with the lowest amounts and 0 grams of trans fat per serving, and remember to avoid foods with partially hydrogenated oil.

Polyunsaturated Fat and Monounsaturated Fat: These are heart-healthy fats and should be consumed more often. As the FDA does not require these fats to be listed on food labels, depending on the food manufacturer, they may or may not be included.

If not listed, figure the amount of unsaturated fat by subtracting the amount of saturated and trans fats from the total fat. In this example, total fat is 8g and saturated fat is 1g, and 8 − 1 = 7; so the remaining 7g are in the form of unsaturated fats.

5. Cholesterol: Guidelines have changed, and there is currently no recommended limit on cholesterol. However, foods high in cholesterol tend to be high in saturated fat, which is a bigger risk factor for heart disease.

6. Sodium: If you have high blood pressure, choose lower-sodium foods, defined as having no more than 140 mg per serving.

7. Total Carbohydrate: This number includes sugar, starch, sugar alcohols, and fiber. Adjust portion sizes based on your carbohydrate consumption goals.

8. Fiber: Its many important functions include blood sugar management, colon health, and reducing cholesterol. Choose and frequently consume foods with at least 3 grams per serving.

9. Total Sugars: This number includes both sugars found naturally in the food product and any added sugars, such as honey, maple syrup, or molasses.

10. Added Sugars: These are sugars that do not occur naturally in the food and have been added to it, such as honey, maple syrup, or molasses. Limit these to meet your nutrient needs while controlling your calorie intake. Too much sugar can lead to weight gain and can spike blood sugar levels.

Nutrition Facts

8 servings per container

Serving size		**2/3 cup (55g)**

Amount per serving

Calories 230

	% Daily Value*
Total Fat 8g	**10%**
Saturated Fat 1g	**5%**
Trans Fat 0g	
Cholesterol 0mg	**0%**
Sodium 160mg	**7%**
Total Carbohydrate 37g	**13%**
Dietary Fiber 4g	**14%**
Total Sugars 12g	
Includes 10g Added Sugars	**20%**
Protein 3g	
Vitamin D 2mcg	10%
Calcium 260mg	20%
Iron 8mg	45%
Potassium 235mg	6%

* The % Daily Value (DV) tells you how much a nutrient in a serving of food contributes to a daily diet. 2,000 calories a day is used for general nutrition advice.

Your best bet is to carefully choose more slow digesting–carbohydrate foods. Keep in mind even these should be eaten in moderation—portion sizes are key. Choose whole fruits about the size of a tennis ball; starchy vegetables such as beans, corn, potatoes, and peas should fill only one-fourth of your plate; and serving sizes of grains, such as oatmeal or brown rice, should be ½ cup.

HYDRATION

Drinking adequate water each day is an important part of any healthy diet. Not only does water keep you well hydrated, but it can also help prevent hyperglycemia, high blood sugars that make the blood thicker and sticky and can increase insulin resistance (the sticky blood makes it even harder for glucose to move through small blood vessels and into the cells). Drinking plenty of water, 10 to 15 cups a day, may help keep blood thinner, meaning glucose can more easily travel into cells where it's needed. Work new habits into your day to help avoid dehydration. Try drinking a glass of water after every bathroom break, infusing water with fresh fruit slices, drinking herbal tea, and drinking a glass of water before each meal.

Sugary beverages, such as soda, sweet tea, lemonade, sports and energy drinks, and juices, are loaded with excessive amounts of sugar and should be consumed rarely. Most only offer empty calories that turn very rapidly into quick-digesting carbohydrates, flooding your bloodstream with too much sugar.

When it comes to drinking alcohol, moderation is key. Women should have only one drink per day, while men should limit themselves to no more than two. Studies show that women may develop alcohol-related problems sooner and at lower drinking levels than men. Keep in mind that women, on average, weigh less than men; women have less water in their bodies than men, leading to a higher blood alcohol concentration, which puts them at greater risk for harm.

Many alcoholic beverages are dehydrating, and some cocktails are quite sugary, again spiking blood sugar. Drink water to prevent dehydration, and never consume alcohol on an empty stomach; it can cause a dangerous drop in blood sugar known as hypoglycemia.

BUILDING A HEALTHY PLATE

When diagnosed with prediabetes, it can be difficult to know where to begin. One of the best ways to start improving your overall food choices is by learning to adjust portion sizes of the foods you eat. The simple plate method is an excellent way to not only eat healthier, well-balanced meals but also manage blood glucose levels. Best of all, there are no special tools required—just a plate. Follow these six simple steps:

1. Imagine a line down the middle of a 9-inch plate. Divide one of the sections in half, creating three sections total.

2. The largest section is for nonstarchy vegetables, such as salad, broccoli, cauliflower, carrots, and tomatoes.

3. In one of the smaller sections, include a healthy starchy food, such as whole-grain bread, brown rice, corn, beans, or potatoes.

4. In the other smaller section, select a healthy lean protein, such as chicken breast, fish, lean meat, eggs, or tofu.

5. Add a serving of fruit and a serving of dairy on the side as your meal plan allows.

6. Complete your meal with a noncalorie beverage, such as water, unsweetened tea, or coffee.

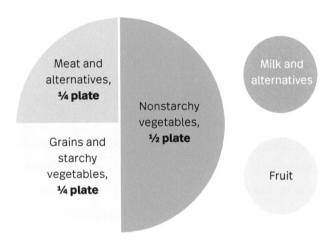

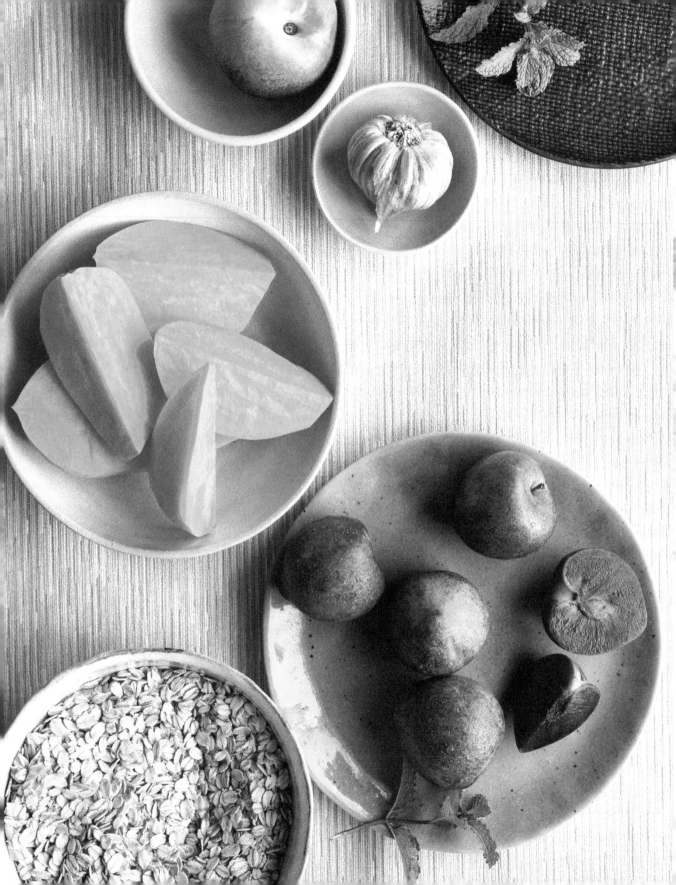

TWO

A Whole-Health Plan

A winning strategy for conquering prediabetes is to start, in whatever way you can, *today*. You have the tools you need to reverse the diagnosis! Prediabetes is progressive, so each day that goes by is a missed opportunity. Many people are unknowingly walking around with prediabetes—and most will eventually be diagnosed with type 2 diabetes. If they had caught it at the prediabetes stage, you can bet they would have done anything to trade the complications and danger of an incurable disease for a reversible and easy-to-treat one.

This chapter focuses on easy ways to incorporate better health habits that will help avoid, or at least slow, the transition to type 2 diabetes. Healthy food choices are an essential component to this, but think of food as just one cog in the wheel of a healthier life plan. Exercise, stress management, and even sleep are also factors that can affect blood glucose.

The Prediabetes Diet

A person's food choices matter—whether or not they have prediabetes. While your focus may be on reversing your diagnosis, adopting an overall healthy diet will also reduce your risk for heart disease, obesity, stroke, and common cancers. That's a win-win for your long-term health.

You may believe avoiding all sugar and carbohydrate-rich foods will become your new normal. But to avoid these foods completely is unrealistic. Instead, focus on changes you can make for the long-term: Carefully monitor portion sizes, and consume fewer sugary foods and beverages. The bulk of your diet should come from nutrient-dense foods—those that provide more nutrients per calorie. For example, compare a kiwi fruit to a handful of gummy bears. Both contain sugar—kiwi has natural sugar, while gummy bears are a manufactured food with added sugar. However, kiwi is also packed with valuable nutrients such as vitamins, minerals, and fiber, while gummy bears basically provide only (empty) calories and little else. No one says you have to eat perfectly, but by frequently filling your plate with nourishing, nutrient-dense foods, you'll be headed toward your best health yet.

RECONSIDER "RULES"

There are many misconceptions or "food rules" of what to eat or avoid. You may have been told to give up all your favorite foods or only eat sugar-free items. Not true. Here's a look at common myths about eating healthy when you have prediabetes.

Myth: You have to give up desserts.
By making modifications, such as having one scoop of ice cream instead of two, eating fruit instead of sugary desserts, or tweaking a favorite recipe by using less sugar, you can still enjoy desserts on occasion.

Myth: You need to eat special diabetic food.
The foods that are good for you are also healthy food choices for the rest of your family. You will simply keep a close eye on controlling the amounts and types of carbohydrates, fat, and protein you eat.

Myth: You must avoid processed foods.
Processed foods are more than just boxed macaroni and cheese, potato chips, and drive-thru hamburgers. The term "processed food" includes any food purposely changed in some way prior to consumption. Many healthy foods

are considered "processed" and are perfectly fine to eat. Minimally processed foods such as bagged spinach, cut vegetables, roasted nuts, canned tuna, or frozen fruits and vegetables are great options to keep on hand.

Myth: You should only choose foods labeled "natural" or "organic."
There is no legal definition of the term "natural," and "organic" has quite a lengthy definition. A cookie could be labeled organic no matter what type of sugar was used, but it should still be eaten in moderation. Organic foods can also carry a high price tag compared to conventionally grown foods; both types provide nutrition, so go with what you can afford and what's realistic for your lifestyle.

Myth: You should only buy food found on the perimeter of the store.
It's true that many healthy foods, such as fruits, vegetables, and fresh meat, are found on the perimeter of grocery stores. But there are plenty of wholesome foods found within the aisles—canned or dried beans, canned tuna or salmon, whole grains such as farro, brown rice, and whole-wheat bread, frozen fruits and vegetables, and nuts and nut butters, to name a few.

HELPFUL AND HEALTHY

Luckily, an overall eating plan for prediabetes is not restrictive, making it easy to follow. If you lean toward more of a Mediterranean-style meal plan or the DASH diet (Dietary Approaches to Stop Hypertension), go for it, as they come with similar principles. In addition, here are other smart, helpful, and healthy guidelines to help stabilize blood sugar.

Stop random eating. No more grabbing a handful of chips or a couple of cookies when you see them.

Use smaller dinner plates. No more than 9 inches in diameter to control portion sizes.

Fill your plate with a combination of foods. Include some carbohydrates, protein, and healthy fat.

Sit down to eat every meal. Sitting helps you focus on your food, enjoying the experience of eating.

Eat slowly. It will help you feel satisfied and lead you to stop eating when you feel full, not stuffed.

Drink water with and between meals. Flavor water with calorie-free add-ins, such as citrus slices, cucumber slices, or a couple of smashed berries.

Eat salad every day. Top salads with a variety of veggies such as cherry tomatoes, sliced mushrooms and carrots, shredded purple cabbage, or diced peppers.

Avoid skipping meals. Eat breakfast, lunch, and dinner.

Read nutrition labels on packaged foods. Pay attention to the serving size and total grams of carbohydrates.

DIETARY RECOMMENDATIONS

Eating healthy for prediabetes is all about making smart food choices and controlling portion size. Focus on choosing whole foods, and you can feel confident you are meeting your nutritional needs. Instead of looking at this as restrictive, refocus your plan to select from among the numerous delicious foods you can eat, including a variety of vegetables, fruits, whole grains, beans, legumes, fish, skinless poultry, lean meat, nuts, and nonfat/low-fat dairy products. You will simply have to limit sugary drinks, sweets, fatty or processed meats, solid fats, and salty or other highly processed foods (and actually, everyone should limit these items!).

Following is a handy guide to help you manage your daily servings of each food. These assume you're consuming either 1,600 or 2,000 calories a day, so your specific needs may vary due to a number of factors including age, activity level, and weight goals.

These dietary recommendations contain today's best scientific advice on the selection of foods for promoting health, preventing disease, and maintaining or losing weight. These recommendations apply to most people and can be a smart way to reach your best health yet. Anyone with a chronic disease or other special nutritional needs should contact a registered dietitian for specific recommendations.

FOOD GROUP	1,600 CALORIES PER DAY	2,000 CALORIES PER DAY	ONE SERVING EQUIVALENT
GRAINS*	6 servings	6 to 8 servings	1 slice bread 1 ounce dry cereal ½ cup cooked rice or pasta (about the size of a baseball)
VEGETABLES	3 to 4 servings	4 to 5 servings	1 cup raw leafy vegetables ½ cup cut raw or cooked vegetables ½ cup vegetable juice
FRUITS	4 servings	4 to 5 servings	1 medium piece of fruit (about the size of a tennis ball) ¼ cup dried fruit ½ cup fresh, frozen, or unsweetened canned fruit ½ cup fruit juice
NONFAT OR LOW-FAT DAIRY	2 to 3 servings	2 to 3 servings	1 cup nonfat or low-fat milk 1 cup nonfat or low-fat yogurt or cottage cheese 1½ ounces nonfat or low-fat cheese
LEAN MEATS, POULTRY, SEAFOOD, EGGS	3 to 6 ounces	Up to 6 ounces	3 ounces cooked meat (size of a deck of cards) 3 ounces grilled fish (size of your palm) 1 egg (no more than 4 per week) 2 egg whites (no limit)—fat is only found in the yolk, not the white
FATS AND OILS	2 servings per day	2 to 3 servings per day	1 teaspoon soft margarine 1 teaspoon vegetable oil 1 tablespoon mayonnaise 1 to 2 tablespoons salad dressing
NUTS, SEEDS, AND LEGUMES	3 to 4 servings per week	4 to 5 servings per week	⅓ cup or 1½ ounces nuts 2 tablespoons peanut or other nut butter 2 tablespoons or ½ ounce seeds ½ cup cooked dried beans or peas
SWEETS	3 or fewer servings per week	5 or fewer servings per week	1 tablespoon sugar 1 tablespoon jam ½ cup sorbet 1 cup lemonade

*At least half of your servings should be whole grains

The Body and Mind

Living well with a condition that could progress into a chronic disease requires taking care of your whole body. In addition to healthy eating, you should nurture several other healthy lifestyle habits to help you become the master of your health. It's like a puzzle: Each piece contributes to the whole picture—if even one piece is missing, the picture is not complete. Work with your health care team to design a prediabetes management plan. You are the expert on you. By setting priorities and goals, you will be protecting your health now and for the future.

GET MOVING

The benefits of physical activity cannot be overstated—for anyone, but especially for those with prediabetes or diabetes. Getting active is a huge part of living healthy while helping lower your blood glucose, and it can be just as important as diet and even medication. If you are not currently exercising on a regular basis, consult your health care provider before you start.

One possible reason you may have developed prediabetes could be inactivity. Many adults find it difficult to fit exercise into their busy lives. For instance, if your job involves prolonged periods of sitting, and then you come home and sit most of the evening, this sets you up for increased insulin resistance.

Specifically for those with prediabetes and diabetes, being physically active is a key part of managing blood glucose. When you are up and moving, your cells become more sensitive to insulin so it can work more efficiently. This helps lower your blood glucose to a more normal range. Other benefits of physical activity include the following:

» Increased energy and endurance throughout the day
» Weight loss and increased muscle tone
» A healthier heart and lower blood pressure
» Restful sleep
» Increased bone strength and, with it, a lower risk of osteoporosis
» Immune system boost
» Lowered cholesterol levels
» Stress management and all the benefits that come with that

The trick to moving more is to find an exercise routine you enjoy and look forward to. Joining a gym or investing in pricey sports equipment is not necessary. A daily 30-minute or longer brisk walk is attainable and convenient for most people. But feel free to explore other activities, such as aerobic exercise, strength training, and flexibility stretches. These can all aid overall health.

CONDITION YOURSELF

You've been learning how and why to eat and exercise to reverse prediabetes. Now let's turn this information into healthy habits.

Habits are automatic behaviors that can make our lives easier, safer, or healthier. For example, locking your doors before going to bed is a spontaneous safety habit. Forming new habits requires understanding the reward, or benefit, of doing so, and takes a little bit of time and practice. To dramatically improve your chances of following through on your desired new habits, try a three-part pattern called the habit loop. This breaks down all habits into three components: *cue*, *routine*, and *reward*. Practiced consistently, they can help solidify a new healthy habit.

Here's an example of a not-so-healthy habit: The *cue* is seeing a fast-food restaurant sign in the distance, the *routine* is pulling up to the drive-thru window to order a chocolate shake, and the *reward* is the delicious chocolatey taste. This can become a habit loop, causing you to repeat the same behavior over and over—even if you know it's bad for you.

By understanding habit loops, you can piggyback them to help form new healthy habits. Let's say you want to set a goal to walk each night after dinner. Piggyback your walk onto the habit of putting the dishes into the dishwasher. The *cue*, then, is loading the dishwasher after dinner. The subsequent walk is your *routine*. The *reward* is having more energy and feeling healthier. Keep this up—the first few times will feel unnatural, but it will change—and eventually you'll have a new healthy habit that's just as ingrained as the unhealthy or spontaneous ones.

Research has shown that forming healthy habits depends on keeping the action simple and consistent. Changes won't happen overnight—it takes about 66 days for any new habit to take hold. Once established, it becomes effortless, and you no longer have to think about it.

SET GOALS

Goal setting is an empowering way of steering yourself in the right direction and working toward establishing regular habits. If you are not sure what to target, ask your doctor what actions would be most beneficial to your health. You can also determine this by asking yourself:

» What do I want to accomplish?
» How will reaching this goal benefit me?

» Will others be involved in helping me reach this goal? Who will support me in my efforts?

» How and where will I carry out this plan?

» What will keep me motivated to keep reaching for my goals?

» What barriers might get in the way of reaching my goals?

Once you decide which areas (healthy eating, exercise, weight loss, sleep, stress management, etc.) need work, you are ready to set specific goals.

The best way to make a goal is to use the SMART goal-setting method. This method brings structure and accountability to your goals and breaks things down into smaller objectives. It sets you up for success and prevents vague, unclear goals (which are more likely to fail). SMART stands for Specific, Measurable, Achievable, Relevant, and Timebound:

(S) **Specific:** Write out clear, concise goals.

(M) **Measurable:** Establish a way to track progress (keep a journal or food diary, use a Fitbit, wear a pedometer).

(A) **Achievable:** Goals should be challenging yet realistic—a too-lofty goal will feel out of reach and lead to giving up too easily.

(R) **Relevant:** Set goals relevant to your overall life plan.

(T) **Timebound:** The goals should have a beginning and an end.

To show you the contrast between a vague goal and a SMART goal, consider these examples:

Vague goal: I will start to exercise by walking more.
SMART goal: I will increase my activity by walking 20 minutes, 3 days a week.

Vague goal: I will start eating breakfast.
SMART goal: I will eat breakfast at 7 a.m. three mornings a week on Monday, Wednesday, and Friday.

THE IMPORTANCE OF SLEEP

A well-rested body is a priceless asset on your health journey. Too many late nights and struggles with falling or remaining asleep can affect your health more than you may know. Sleep gives your body a chance to rest and recover. Your organs, muscles, and even your immune system are able to remain strong and healthy when you have a good night's sleep. Even your weight is affected by sleep, or lack thereof, because insufficient shut-eye negatively affects the hormones that influence your appetite (ghrelin, the hunger hormone, and leptin, a hormone that makes you feel full).

Several studies have also found that poor sleep quality and quantity affects glucose metabolism and can increase the risk of prediabetes. Sleepless nights can be a form of chronic stress on your body, and added stress can result in higher blood sugar levels. A lack of sleep reduces your body's sensitivity to insulin, leading to an increased amount of sugar in your bloodstream. On top of everything, when blood sugar is higher than normal, your kidneys try to remove it from the body by increasing urination—so you might experience a higher frequency of nighttime bathroom visits, resulting in inconsistent sleep patterns. Controlling your blood sugar with healthier eating, exercise, and stress management can help you get the rest your body needs.

To get a better night's sleep, here are a few tips from the National Sleep Foundation:

- » Have a bedtime routine: Go to bed and get up the next morning at the same time every day.
- » Keep blinds and curtains open during the day to help regulate your sleep-wake cycle.
- » Get outdoors during the day.
- » Exercise daily.
- » Avoid using electronic devices 1 to 2 hours before bedtime.
- » Avoid eating big meals at night that can result in heartburn and poor digestion.
- » Avoid alcohol or too many liquids before bed to avoid frequent bathroom trips.
- » Sleep in a cool room (60 to 67 degrees Fahrenheit), free from any light or distractions.

The Kitchen

Your kitchen is the heart of your home and the perfect place to focus your attention toward long-term healthy eating habits. When your cupboards, pantry, refrigerator, and freezer are stocked with healthy foods, meal preparation will be a breeze. Begin to purge not-so-healthy foods, such as ice cream, soda, cookies, or sugary cereals, making room for nutritious options. These lifestyle changes are invaluable for controlling blood sugar, maintaining a healthy body weight, and serving delicious, healthy meals you and your family will appreciate.

To help you identify which foods to keep on hand, here's a look at basic staples of healthy eating. No need to run out and buy every single item listed—instead, each week, try to add a few foods you don't currently keep stocked. Having these inexpensive, ready-to-go basics for making meals will simplify your life while enhancing your health.

Foods to Stock

When you look into your cupboards or pantry, you should see foods that are high in fiber and protein and low in sugar, salt, and saturated fats. Following is a list of foods that meet the criteria:

» Canned or dried beans, lentils, or split peas
» Canned refried beans, fat-free
» Canned broths, low-sodium
» Canned vegetables, low-sodium or no-salt-added
» Canned tomatoes, tomato sauce, and tomato paste, no-salt-added
» Canned fruits, unsweetened or packed-in-own-juice
» Canned tuna, salmon, or chicken, water-packed
» Dried fruit
» Healthy oils, such as olive or canola, and nonstick cooking spray
» Natural nut butters such as natural peanut or almond butter
» Nuts and peanuts, unsalted
» Old-fashioned or quick-cooking oatmeal (not instant)

» Popcorn
» Potatoes and sweet potatoes
» Seeds: chia, flax, hemp, pumpkin, sunflower
» Spaghetti sauce
» Vinegars, such as red or white wine
» Whole-grain cereals, with at least 5 grams of fiber per serving
» Whole grains, such as barley, buckwheat, bulgur, brown rice, farro, quinoa, and wheat berries
» Whole-wheat bread (100 percent), with at least 2 grams of fiber per serving
» Whole-wheat crackers, with at least 2 grams of fiber per serving
» Whole-wheat pasta
» Whole-wheat tortillas

Foods to Remove

Now that you know which foods should be in your pantry, here is a (short!) list of foods to remove. Many of these highly processed foods are sources of unhealthy saturated or trans fats, high levels of sodium, refined low-fiber grains, or added sugars.

- » Cake or brownie mixes
- » Candy
- » Creamy salad dressings
- » Granola bars
- » Jams and jelly

- » Sugary beverages, such as soda, sports drinks, lemonade, or sweetened tea mixes
- » Sugary breakfast cereals (those with more than 6 grams of sugar per serving)

REFRIGERATOR AND FREEZER

Thanks to modern-day appliances, we have the luxury of eating a wide variety of nutritious foods year-round. When you open your refrigerator or freezer doors, you should see the following healthy foods:

Foods to Stock

Here are a few items to keep in your fridge and freezer for go-to healthy meal solutions:

- » Eggs
- » Fresh fruits and vegetables, a variety
- » Fresh herbs
- » Frozen edamame
- » Frozen fruits, unsweetened
- » Frozen vegetables, without sauce
- » Greek yogurt, nonfat or low-fat
- » Hummus
- » Leafy greens, such as arugula, kale, or spinach

- » Lean animal proteins, such as beef, chicken, fish, pork, and turkey
- » Leftovers or cooked extras, such as beans, rice, or quinoa
- » Low-fat cheese, including Babybel, cottage, Parmesan, and string
- » Mustard, Dijon
- » Nonfat or low-fat milk and nondairy milk alternatives, such as almond or soy milk

Foods to Remove

On the flip side, there are many foods and beverages that can and should be removed from a healthy diet. Avoid stocking your fridge or freezer with the following:

- » Alcoholic beverages
- » Butter or margarine, stick form
- » Creamy salad dressings
- » Fish sticks
- » Frozen french fries and pizza

- » Gourmet ice cream
- » Processed meats, such as bologna, hot dogs, or sausage
- » Soda

SATISFYING CRAVINGS

Everyone experiences food cravings. The trick is to manage them before they become a problem. When food cravings strike, determine whether it's true hunger or simply appetite. Hunger is physiological: You haven't eaten for many hours, and physically, you feel hungry, in which case it's okay to choose a healthy snack. Appetite is more psychological: You just ate a big meal and are full, but psychologically you still crave a sweet dessert.

Emotional triggers also cause cravings. Feelings of anger, frustration, worry, loneliness, sadness, or even boredom can lead to using food as a source of comfort. Food cravings also result from lack of sleep or needing an energy boost or to calm anxiety.

If food cravings are ruling your life, here are some steps to help kick them to the curb:

» Create more well-balanced meals and snacks to keep handy.

» Distract yourself—take a walk, call a friend, listen to music.

» Get adequate sleep.

» Give in, but choose healthy alternatives.

» Identify your triggers, and remove them if you can.

» Limit exposure to trigger foods.

» Practice recognizing the difference between hunger and appetite. Wait 10 minutes or drink a tall glass of water to see if the craving subsides.

Keep these healthy go-to snacks on hand for when cravings hit:

» Sliced carrots, cucumbers, and bell peppers with guacamole or hummus for dipping

» ¼ to ½ cup dry-roasted chickpeas or nuts

» Small apple or pear with nut butter

» ½ cup cottage cheese with fresh or frozen berries

» Small handful of almonds with grapes

» 2 cups popcorn with ¼ cup peanuts

EQUIPMENT ESSENTIALS

Now it's time to outfit your kitchen with the tools to make meal prep a cinch. First, take an inventory of the equipment you already have. Decide which to keep and which to sell or donate—for example, plan to sell that deep-fat fryer! Here is a list of essentials to make healthy, delicious meals easier and faster:

» Blender or food processor
» Cutting boards for different food groups
» Electric pressure cooker, such as Instant Pot, or slow cooker
» Food scale for portion control
» Hand chopper for veggies
» Measuring spoons and cups
» Meat thermometer for ensuring food safety
» Microwave
» Oil mister
» Quality set of sharp knives
» Stand mixer
» Steamer basket
» Vegetable spiralizer
» Well-stocked spice rack

ABOUT THE RECIPES

You'll see the following labels used in part 2, to guide you in selecting the best recipes for your needs and make preparing healthy meals easy and fuss-free.

» **5 Ingredient:** These recipes contain five ingredients or fewer (not including salt, pepper, oil, and water).
» **30 Minutes or Less:** These recipes can be on the table in a half hour or less, including prep and cooking time.
» **Dairy Free:** These recipes are free of milk, yogurt, cheese, and other dairy-containing ingredients.
» **Gluten Free:** These recipes are free of gluten and gluten-containing foods.
» **Nut Free:** These recipes contain no tree nuts or peanuts.
» **One Pot:** The entire recipe can be prepared in one cooking vessel.
» **Vegetarian:** These recipes contain no meat or meat products.
» **Vegan:** These recipes are free of meat, dairy, or other animal products.

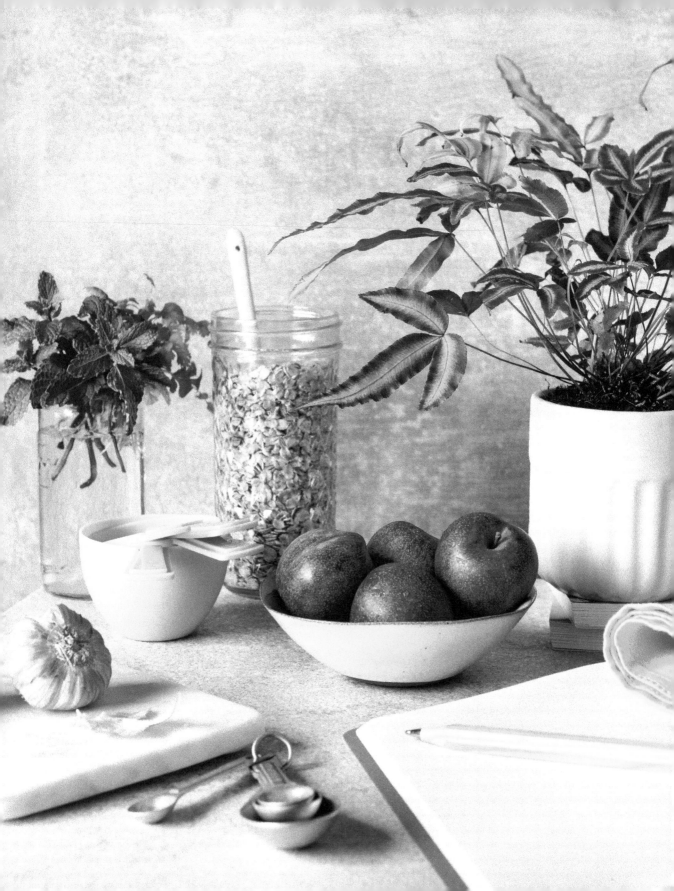

THREE

A 2-Week Action and Meal Plan

Ready, set, go! This chapter will get you started with a doable, actionable 2-week meal and activity plan. Once you see how easy it is to cook healthy meals, add some daily physical activity, and practice healthy habits, you'll be well on your way toward conquering prediabetes.

Having a 2-week meal plan helps take the guesswork out of what to eat. For 14 days, you will have a specific, effective (and delicious!) plan for breakfast, lunch, and dinner. This book contains 75 tasty, prediabetes-friendly recipes to give you plenty of options. This allows you to customize the menu and makes it easier to stick to the plan.

I know life gets busy. Rushed mornings, work all day, come home late to fix dinner—it's hard to get it all done. I also know it's not practical to cook three meals a day. That's why many of the recipes are designed for easy, grab-and-go weekday breakfasts and lunches. With some helpful suggestions on meal prep for the week ahead, you'll have everything you need for success.

To get you moving more and sleeping better, you will also find an activity plan offering realistic activities and tips to help you form new habits and routines. Don't worry if your current exercise regimen is nonexistent—anyone can add some healthy movement to their day.

Finally, you will learn actionable tips on how to stay on track during holidays, social events, or while on vacation. You have everything you need at your fingertips, so let's get the ball rolling and take action today.

Week 1

A key part of controlling blood glucose is eating healthy foods every day. You don't have to stop eating the foods you like, but this is your opportunity to begin a new journey toward creating healthy meals for you and your family. When you follow the 2-week meal plan, you'll learn how to adapt to a new way of cooking, eating, and thinking about food and your health. But this isn't a crash diet or a restrictive cleanse; it's just easy, good-for-you food.

This action plan breaks down into three easy steps: a prep plan, a meal plan, and an activity plan. You'll form new healthy habits by repeating them most days, if not every day, of the week. When made a regular part of your daily routine, they will become a part of what you do for years to come as you work to get, and remain, healthy.

WEEK 1 PREP PLAN

Meal prepping, or simply "meal prep," has become a popular cooking trend. It involves preparing food a day or more in advance to help reduce eating out or reliance on highly processed foods and instead enjoying tasty, healthier, home-cooked meals. You'll be amazed how quickly these dishes can come together. Here are a few things you can do to prep for the week.

Sunday:

Berry-Oat Breakfast Bars (page 52): Make this recipe and store in a covered container. They'll keep for up to 5 days.

Vegetable Chowder (page 76): Make and keep refrigerated in a covered container.

Tuesday evening:

Egg and Veggie Breakfast Cups (page 62): Chop the veggies and keep refrigerated in an airtight container until ready to use.

Turkey Meat Loaf (page 87): Prep all ingredients and refrigerate in separate containers.

Wednesday evening:

Make the **Mushroom Gravy** (page 115) to go with the Turkey Meat Loaf. While it cooks, chop the veggies for the **Salmon and Veggie Bake** (page 82). Refrigerate the veggies in a covered container.

Peach Muesli Bake (page 57): Soak the oats in milk for about 20 minutes to cut your cooking time in half.

Friday evening:

Breakfast Tostada (page 63): Bake the corn tortillas the night before.

Saturday:

Make the **Whole-Grain Pancakes** (page 55), keep refrigerated in a resealable plastic bag for up to 5 days, and reheat in the toaster on Sunday—or any—morning.

	BREAKFAST	LUNCH	DINNER
MON	**Berry-Oat Breakfast Bars** (page 52)	**Vegetable Chowder** (page 76)	**Herb Roasted Chicken Breast** (page 86); **Quinoa Pilaf** (page 109)
TUE	Leftover **Berry-Oat Breakfast Bars**	Cut up leftover chicken and place on a bed of leafy greens.	**Butternut Squash and Mushroom Lasagna** (page 78)
WED	**Egg and Veggie Breakfast Cups** (page 62)	Plain nonfat Greek yogurt with fresh fruit; baby carrots with hummus	**Turkey Meat Loaf** (page 87) with **Mushroom Gravy** (page 115)
THU	**Peach Muesli Bake** (page 57); plain nonfat Greek yogurt	Leftover **Egg and Veggie Breakfast Cups**	**Salmon and Veggie Bake** (page 82)
FRI	Leftover **Peach Muesli Bake**	Leftover **Turkey Meat Loaf**	**Margherita Pizza** (page 70); side salad with **Balsamic Vinaigrette** (page 113)
SAT	**Breakfast Tostada** (page 63); fresh strawberries	Add leftover salmon to a bed of lettuce with chopped celery, diced bell pepper, and shredded carrots	**Chicken Zoodle Soup** (page 84)
SUN	**Whole-Grain Pancakes** (page 55); fresh fruit	Make a lunch using any leftovers from the week.	Leftover **Chicken Zoodle Soup**

Treat yourself to dessert twice this week: Try **Easy Berry Sorbet** (page 129) on Tuesday and **Roasted Spiced Pears** (page 133) on Saturday.

SNACK OPTIONS

When it comes to snacking, foods high in sugar or with added fats may come to mind, but there are many healthier options that can support proper nutrition and help keep you fueled for the day. Although there are no set rules, a snack or two per day can help most people manage hunger and maintain blood sugar levels. Snacks can definitely be part of a healthy lifestyle, but be mindful of portion sizes and the number of snacks you eat each day. Here are some ideas:

» ¼ cup dried fruit and nut mix

» 1 small apple or orange (size of a tennis ball)

» 3 cups unbuttered popcorn

» ¼ cup hummus with 1 cup fresh cut veggies, such as green bell peppers, carrots, broccoli, cucumber, celery, or cauliflower

» ¼ cup cottage cheese and ½ cup canned (no-sugar-added) or fresh fruit

» 2 tablespoons peanut butter with apple or banana slices

» 1 hard-boiled egg with 1 slice whole-grain toast

» 6 ounces fruit-flavored nonfat Greek yogurt

» Baked pita chips (10) with 2 tablespoons hummus

» 5 whole-wheat crackers and 1 string cheese

» 8 ounces low-fat milk with ¼ cup almonds (or walnuts, cashews, pistachios)

» Reduced-fat cheese and apple slices or grapes

» ½ peanut butter sandwich on whole-grain bread

» Vegetable juice or tomato juice with almonds or reduced-fat cheese

WEEK 1 ACTIVITY PLAN

The importance of physical activity cannot be emphasized enough for treating prediabetes. Not only can it help you lose extra pounds, it's also good for increasing insulin sensitivity, as well as for your heart and overall health. If you have been inactive for a while, this plan will help ease you into a more active lifestyle. The activities suggested are meant to become part of your current routine (such as gardening or playing with your children) as well as manageable and fun—before you know it, you'll be devoting more minutes each day toward physical activity.

A good night's sleep is another "activity" that's part of your improved health plan. Sleep is the body's chance to restore and repair itself in all aspects, including maintenance of the immune system and the body's metabolic functions. Poor sleep affects diabetes by triggering hormones contributing to weight gain and, thereby, increasing the risk of type 2 diabetes. When sleep is disrupted or insufficient, it can lead to poorly controlled diabetes. Luckily, there are many steps you can take to get a better night's sleep.

WEEK 1 ACTIVITY TIPS

Starting a fitness routine is easy; sticking with it is hard. When we don't perceive immediate results our initial enthusiasm disappears, or we get busy and discard our commitment. Yet many people do manage to make exercise a lifelong habit. What's their secret?

» The first "secret" is to start with a variety of activities to choose from—walking, weight lifting, bicycling, tennis, aerobics, and yoga are good options. This ensures an enjoyable experience to look forward to, no matter the weather or how you're feeling.

» Second, make it a nonnegotiable priority. Schedule it in your calendar and do not reschedule it. This is your time.

» Third, work on your sleep. Establishing a pre-bedtime routine, a.k.a. practicing good "sleep hygiene," may help you fall and stay asleep until morning. Again, just like establishing a fitness routine, it takes time to develop sleep habits that stick. Try to stay on schedule by going to bed and waking up at the same time each day—even on weekends.

The following plan contains suggestions for incorporating easy activity into your everyday life. Start small and build throughout the week. If you feel confident, fold some of the previous activities into as many days throughout the week as you can. At the end of the week, you'll have a good idea of the kinds of activities that work best for your fitness goals and lifestyle—and you can make them a part of your regular routine.

	MORNING	MIDDAY	AFTERNOON/EVENING
MON	**Stretch:** After getting out of bed, stretch for 5 minutes.	**Walk:** Take two laps around your home or office.	**Sleep:** Power down from all electronics 1 hour before bedtime.
TUE	**Hydrate:** Within 15 minutes of getting up, drink an 8-ounce glass of water.	**Walk:** Warm up with gentle stretching, then walk for 10 to 15 minutes.	**Sleep:** Set your thermostat between 60 and 67 degrees Fahrenheit before going to bed. This increases natural instincts to sleep, releases melatonin, and improves sleep quality.
WED	**Hydrate:** Aim to drink at least four 8-ounce glasses of water today.	**Walk:** Every hour, get up and walk for 5 minutes. **Cardio:** Take the stairs.	**Yoga/Sleep:** Do 5 minutes of beginner's yoga before bedtime (see page 39)
THU	**Stretch:** After getting out of bed, stretch for 10 minutes. **Hydrate:** Aim to drink at least five 8-ounce glasses of water today.	**Cardio:** Park at the far end of a parking lot, whether a shopping center or at work, and walk briskly to the entrance.	**Walk:** During commercial breaks, walk in place or do laps around the room. **Sleep:** Avoid drinking any caffeinated beverages at least 4 hours before bedtime.
FRI	**Stretch:** After getting out of bed, stretch for 10 minutes. **Hydrate:** Aim to drink at least five 8-ounce glasses of water today. Try fruit-infused water for extra flavor.	**Move while sitting:** At work or home, do knee lifts, alternating knees; leg extensions, alternating extending one leg straight and then back down; and calf raises, keeping the balls of your feet on the floor while lifting heels up and down.	**Weights:** Lift light dumbbells (1 to 5 pounds), or other heavy objects, for 5 minutes. **Sleep:** Practice having the same bedtime and wakeup time each day.
SAT	**Balance:** Practice walking heel to toe in a straight line or standing on one leg at a time for at least 5 seconds **Hydrate:** Aim to drink at least six 8-ounce glasses of water.	**Exercise:** Put on music and dance for 15 to 20 minutes, or take a walk or hike on a nature trail.	**Yoga/Sleep:** Do 5 minutes of mindful breathing before bedtime (see page 39).
SUN	**Balance:** Practice walking backward or sideways. **Hydrate:** Aim to drink at least six 8-ounce glasses of water today.	**Walk:** Warm up with gentle stretching, then walk briskly for 20 minutes at a mall or park.	**Weights:** Lift light weights (1 to 5 pounds), or other heavy objects, for 5 to 10 minutes. **Sleep:** Practice having your last meal or snack at least 2 hours before bedtime.

GETTING STARTED WITH YOGA

A wonderful thing about yoga is that it can be practiced in the comfort of your home. Here are a few tips to create your own private studio space and try some beginner poses:

Choose a quiet, uncluttered space. It doesn't have to be a large area. Use a yoga mat or blanket for cushioning.

Start with 5- to 10-minute blocks of time. Gradually increase as you feel ready.

Begin with the basics. As your skills improve, consider expanding your yoga poses or joining a class to further enhance your skills.

Choose a time of day that suits your schedule. This will keep you motivated and invigorated.

Here are 3 examples of beginner yoga positions:

Child's Pose: Kneel on the floor, knees apart. Bend forward, letting your belly rest between your thighs, and rest your forehead on the floor while reaching your arms out in front of you. Feel a gentle stretch in your lower back.

Supine Twist: Lying on your back, bring your arms out to the sides in a T, palms down. Bring your knees up to your chest, then slowly lower them to your right side to touch the floor, twisting the lower back. Turn your head to look at your left hand, keeping your shoulders on the floor. Breathe and hold the pose for 10 to 15 seconds. Roll back to center and bring your knees to your chest. Repeat on the opposite side.

Mindful breathing: Lie on the floor on your back. Place one hand on your abdomen and the other hand on your chest. Close your eyes and take slow, deep breaths. Let your body relax completely.

Week 2

Good job—you made it through Week 1! You are doing great; you can do this! The first week should have given you a good idea of the lifestyle that will help you overcome prediabetes. Practicing meal prep, eating more healthy meals, and developing healthy exercise and sleep habits are all parts of the good-health puzzle. If you're feeling somewhat overwhelmed by the changes, that's normal. It always feels different when we make progress. Tell yourself, "Small but steady changes will help me reach my goals."

Now, it's time to begin Week 2. These next seven days are a continuation of what you've learned in Week 1. You'll make more delicious recipes and build upon your new routines—drinking more water, increasing activity, and practicing good sleep hygiene. Before you know it, you'll have more energy and feel your best yet.

WEEK 2 PREP PLAN

By now, you should see the benefits of meal prepping. It can save time and money, allows for better portion control, improves your multitasking skills, and lets you get more done with less effort. Healthy eating is easier when meals and snacks are prepped and on hand, making unhealthy eating less likely to tempt you. Before you know it, meal planning and prepping will be a natural part of your lifestyle.

Saturday/Sunday:

Make a batch of **Whole-Grain Breakfast Cookies** (page 53). Store in a tightly covered container, or freeze in reseal-able bags and thaw before eating.

Having a healthy prepared snack ready to eat is easy when you prep either **Dark Chocolate Drops** (page 128) or **Almond Power Balls** (page 132). Store separately in tightly covered containers.

Monday/Tuesday:

Buy preshredded carrots and cabbage from the produce section of your grocery store for **Asian-Style Chicken Wraps** (page 89).

Wednesday evening:

Consider prepping **Cucumber Salad** (page 102) 2 to 3 days before serving—keeping it refrigerated in an airtight container.

WEEK 2 MEAL PLAN

	BREAKFAST	LUNCH	DINNER
MON	Steel-Cut Oatmeal Bowl with Fruit and Nuts (page 58)	Lentil and Vegetable Soup (page 73)	Baked Parmesan-Crusted Halibut (page 83)
TUE	Whole-Grain Breakfast Cookies (page 53)	Leftover Lentil and Vegetable Soup	Spaghetti with Chickpea and Mushroom Marinara (page 80)
WED	Leftover Whole-Grain Breakfast Cookies	Melt turkey, apple slices, and Cheddar on whole-wheat bread in the toaster oven	Asian-Style Chicken Wraps (page 89)
THU	Spinach and Cheese Quiche (page 61)	Leftover Asian-Style Chicken Wraps	Flank Steak with Chimichurri (page 96)
FRI	Leftover Spinach and Cheese Quiche	Chickpea, Tomato, and Kale Soup (page 72)	Herb-Crusted Pork Tenderloin (page 95) and Cucumber Salad (page 102)
SAT	Sweet Potato Hash with Eggs (page 65)	Veggie bowl with spinach, sliced avocado, walnuts, cucumbers, red bell peppers, and chickpeas	Simple Salmon Burgers (page 81)
SUN	Leftover Sweet Potato Hash with Eggs	Make a lunch using any leftovers from the week.	Black Bean Soup (page 74)

Treat yourself to dessert twice this week: Try **Sweet Potato Cake** (page 135) on Monday and **Tropical Fruit Salad with Coconut Milk** (page 122) on Thursday or Friday.

INGREDIENT SWAPS

When it comes to food, small changes can make a big impact—as in swapping out not-so-healthy ingredients. Best of all, you can do this without sacrificing flavor. Here are some simple swaps to try.

INGREDIENT	HEALTHIER SWAPS
ALL-PURPOSE FLOUR	Whole-wheat pastry flour
BACON	Canadian bacon, turkey bacon, or vegetarian bacon
BROTH	Reduced- or low-sodium broths
BUTTER	Unsweetened applesauce, mashed banana or avocado, olive oil, or cooking spray
CANNED VEGETABLES	Low- or no-salt canned or frozen vegetables without sauce
FRENCH FRIES	Carrot, sweet potato, or zucchini fries
GROUND BEEF	Extra-lean ground round beef, ground chicken, or turkey
HEAVY CREAM	Evaporated skim milk
MAYONNAISE	Mashed avocado or plain nonfat Greek yogurt
PASTA	Lots of nonstarchy veggies, such as broccoli, mushrooms, spinach, tomatoes, yellow squash, or zucchini
PIZZA CRUST	Thin-crust, flatbread, or cauliflower pizza crust
SALT IN RECIPES	Fresh or dried herbs and spices, salt-free seasonings
SALT ON VEGETABLES	Freshly squeezed lemon juice or vinegar
SOUR CREAM	Reduced-fat sour cream or plain nonfat Greek yogurt
SOY SAUCE	Reduced-sodium or light soy sauce
SPAGHETTI	Spaghetti squash or spiralized zucchini
SUGAR	Sugar substitute blend for baking, or cut regular sugar amounts by 30 to 50 percent
WHITE BREAD	100 percent whole-wheat bread
WHITE RICE	Barley, brown rice, lentils, quinoa, or whole-wheat couscous
WHOLE MILK	Skim, 1%, or 2% milk

WEEK 2 ACTIVITY PLAN

This week, you'll be improving and building upon the work you put in last week. As you tried the various suggestions in Week 1, you probably learned which types of activities worked best for you—from both a fitness perspective and a routine perspective. Remember that incorporating activity—any type of activity—into your day and making it part of your routine is just as important as the activity itself. So pay attention to what works for you, and make substitutions as you figure out the best fit into your lifestyle. Keep trying new things, push yourself to increase the time devoted to your chosen activities, and you will slowly develop new healthy habits. You may even find that Week 2 is just that much easier than Week 1, now that you've made a start.

WEEK 2 ACTIVITY TIPS

It's making activity a part of your routine—and a nonnegotiable priority, as mentioned in Week 1—that is the obstacle for so many. Here are a few things to try to overcome these hurdles.

» Start your day with exercise. If you can include some form of movement within the first hour after waking up, you can avoid unexpected things popping up later in the day to sabotage your routine.

» Reward yourself for achieving certain fitness goals. Buy yourself some new seasonal activewear once you've walked consistently for 2 straight weeks, or splurge on that new bowling ball after being active for a month.

» When it comes to sleep habits, avoid nicotine and caffeine, which are stimulants, at least 4 to 6 hours before bedtime.

» Creating a comfy, quiet bedroom also helps make the atmosphere peaceful and restful. This doesn't necessarily mean redecorating—simply powering down all electronics at least 1 hour before going to bed can greatly improve your sleep quality.

	MORNING	MIDDAY	AFTERNOON/EVENING
MON	**Stretch:** After getting out of bed, stretch for 10 minutes. **Hydrate:** Aim to drink at least seven 8-ounce glasses of water today.	**Walk:** Take a 15- to 20-minute walk over your lunch hour. **Cardio:** Take the stairs at least twice today.	**Sleep:** Read a book or take a warm shower or bath 30 to 60 minutes before bedtime to feel sleepy.
TUE	**Walk:** Stand up and walk every time you talk on the phone today. **Hydrate:** Aim to drink at least seven 8-ounce glasses of water today.	**Balance:** Practice standing on one leg for at least 10 seconds, or practice walking heel to toe in a straight line.	**Weights:** Lift light weights (1 to 5 pounds), or other heavy objects, for 10 to 15 minutes. **Sleep:** Keep lights dim 30 to 60 minutes before going to bed.
WED	**Stretch:** After getting out of bed, stretch for 10 minutes. **Hydrate:** Aim to drink at least eight 8-ounce glasses of water today.	**Walk:** Take a 20- to 30-minute walk today; do gentle stretches afterward.	**Sleep:** Create a quiet environment in your bedroom—remove the TV and use white noise, such as a fan, to induce sleep.
THU	**Stand more:** Gradually build up to standing for at least 15 minutes for every hour seated. **Hydrate:** Aim to drink at least eight 8-ounce glasses of water today.	**Move while sitting:** At work or home, do knee lifts, alternating knees; leg extensions, alternating extending one leg straight and then back down; and calf raises, keeping the balls of your feet on the floor while lifting heels up and down.	**Weights:** Lift light weights (1 to 5 pounds), or other heavy objects, for 10 to 15 minutes. **Yoga/Sleep:** Do 5 minutes of beginner's yoga before bedtime (see page 39).
FRI	**Stretch:** After getting out of bed, stretch for 15 minutes. **Hydrate:** Aim to drink at least eight 8-ounce glasses of water today.	**Walk:** Take a 20- to 30-minute walk today. **Cardio:** Take two flights of stairs or walk uphill.	**Sleep:** Keep a gratitude journal where you write down 3 things you are grateful for before bedtime at least 3 times a week.
SAT	**Balance:** Practice walking backward and sideways. **Hydrate:** Aim to drink at least eight 8-ounce glasses of water today.	**Exercise:** Take a leisurely bike ride, put on music and dance, or walk/hike on a nature trail for 20 to 30 minutes	**Stretch:** Do gentle stretching for 10 minutes. **Sleep:** Keep your bedroom as dark as possible at night.
SUN	**Balance:** Practice standing on one leg with eyes closed for 5 seconds. **Hydrate:** Aim to drink at least eight 8-ounce glasses of water today.	**Walk:** Walk your dog or take a brisk walk around your neighborhood for at least 20 minutes.	**Stretch:** Do gentle stretching for 10 minutes. **Sleep:** Before bedtime, write down 3 things you are grateful for.

Week 3 and Beyond

Congratulations! You've been working hard at establishing, and now maintaining, your goals toward eating healthier and becoming more physically active. Likely you have experienced improvements in several areas—weight loss, increased energy and motivation, and overall feeling healthier. You've begun your journey of fighting back prediabetes while reducing the risks of other diseases. This is your lifelong plan for healthy eating and regular activity.

LONG-TERM PAYOFF

It's important to be on the lookout for possible roadblocks to long-term success, even though everything may be going smoothly right now. To keep yourself on track and turn what you've learned in two weeks into lifelong habits, here are things to keep in mind:

» Set realistic goals. Make them achievable within a reasonable amount of time to keep you from getting discouraged if they are not met. Small achievements and positive results motivate further good habits.

» Remember this is your health we're talking about, not some abstract concept. Be honest with yourself about what motivates you, and use that to stay committed.

» Out of sight, out of mind. Ditch the unhealthy foods from your pantry and refrigerator to remove temptation.

» Progress is slow and steady. Forgive yourself if you have a bad day, and start fresh tomorrow. One bad choice does not a failure make.

» Practice mindful eating. Savor the aromas, flavors, and textures of your food. Slow down and let your body have a chance to tell you it's full. Swap your clean plate club membership for the healthy plate club.

» Keep a food and exercise journal. It's fun to look back and see what recipes you've tried that are now new favorites and look for patterns and changes in your activity log.

BACKUP OPTIONS

Inevitably, things will go awry. This also applies to your meal plan. The power goes out. You forget to thaw something. You forget to bring your lunch to work. You discover spoiled produce. Life happens. That's why a good backup plan is nice to have. Here are some foolproof and healthy ideas:

» Stock up on nutrient-rich foods with a long shelf life that can easily become delicious, healthy meals. Canned tuna can be made into tuna salad. Canned or dried beans can be added to soups, stews, or even meat loaf as a good protein source. Quick-cooking brown rice, oatmeal, whole-grain pasta, and whole-grain cereals are high in fiber and important B vitamins that help

HOLIDAYS, VACATIONS, AND EVENTS

At home you're in control of making meals and snacks. But invariably situations will arise—holidays, vacations, social events—and you won't know what to eat. Don't panic. With some advance planning, you can have success, even away from home.

When eating out:

» Instead of breaded or fried foods, choose broiled, roasted, grilled, or steamed.

» Ask the waiter not to bring bread or tortilla chips to the table.

» Choose a side salad or double order of vegetables instead of french fries.

» Make a meal out of a salad or soup.

» Ask for sauces and dressings on the side, and use sparingly. Avoid creamy dressings such as ranch or Thousand Island, and use an oil and vinegar dressing instead.

» Most restaurants serve large portions; request a take-home container and eat only half your meal.

» Avoid buffet-style restaurants.

» Split dessert with a friend or family member or have a piece of fruit.

When on vacation:

» Follow the same guidelines as when eating out.

» Eat three meals a day with 1 to 2 snacks.

» For breakfast, have a good source of protein such as eggs, Greek yogurt, or oatmeal with nuts. Skip sugary pastries, donuts, and juices.

you feel energized, while peanut or other nut butters are easily made into a wholesome sandwich.

» Keep at least a couple of fruits and veggies with a long refrigeration life on hand, such as apples, grapes, carrots, or peppers. Frozen fruits and veggies can last even longer and reduce waste.

» Eggs are always good for a quick, versatile, and filling high-protein meal.

» Dairy foods, such as milk, string cheese, and Greek yogurt, are perfect for providing essential calcium and vitamin D.

» Nuts, seeds, and dried fruit mixed together are an appetizing, nourishing, and quick fix to add to any meal.

» Keep healthy snacks on hand at your hotel—choose fruit, string cheese, baby carrots, peanut butter, nuts, or hummus.

Holidays and special occasions:

» Plan ahead for any special event. If possible, know what type of food will be served and plan to choose more vegetables and lean proteins (eggs, chicken, fish, or beans).

» Bring a dish to share that you know you will enjoy.

» Don't skip meals before the event. To avoid overeating, have a small but filling snack an hour before the occasion, such as apple slices with peanut butter or a small salad with lots of veggies.

» Stay hydrated throughout the day; drinking more water can reduce sugar and calorie intake.

» Pay attention to portions. Take only small amounts of the foods you really want to eat. Eat slowly.

» Move away from the food table.

» Keep dessert portions small, and skip extra toppings.

» Fit in more physical activity on the day of a special occasion.

If you drink alcohol:

» Know that alcohol can lower your blood glucose level, affecting you up to 24 hours after drinking.

» Never drink on an empty stomach.

» Choose lower-calorie options: light beer, dry wines (they have less sugar), or spritzers. Make mixed drinks with diet soda or seltzer water instead of sugary sodas or juices.

THE
RECIPES

Just by reading this far, you've come a long way in promoting and protecting your health. That is a feat in and of itself! Part 1 has given you the information you need about prediabetes to move forward and tackle it head-on. You've learned the role of nutrition, how to read a label, what foods to buy, what a whole-health plan looks like, why exercise is important, how to get moving, and the importance of sleep. That is a great deal to contemplate. You now have the knowledge and motivation to defeat prediabetes once and for all. You've got this.

Part 2 will arm you further, and it's where things get fun—with delicious recipes for you and your family. Let these 75 easy and tempting recipes help make this journey toward good health a reality. From mouthwatering main dishes to savory sides, and even delectable (but healthier) desserts, you will use these simple-to-prepare recipes over and over again. Most recipes also include tips to make cooking a breeze. Get ready to bring out your inner master chef by preparing and eating the simple, delicious foods that will help you reverse prediabetes.

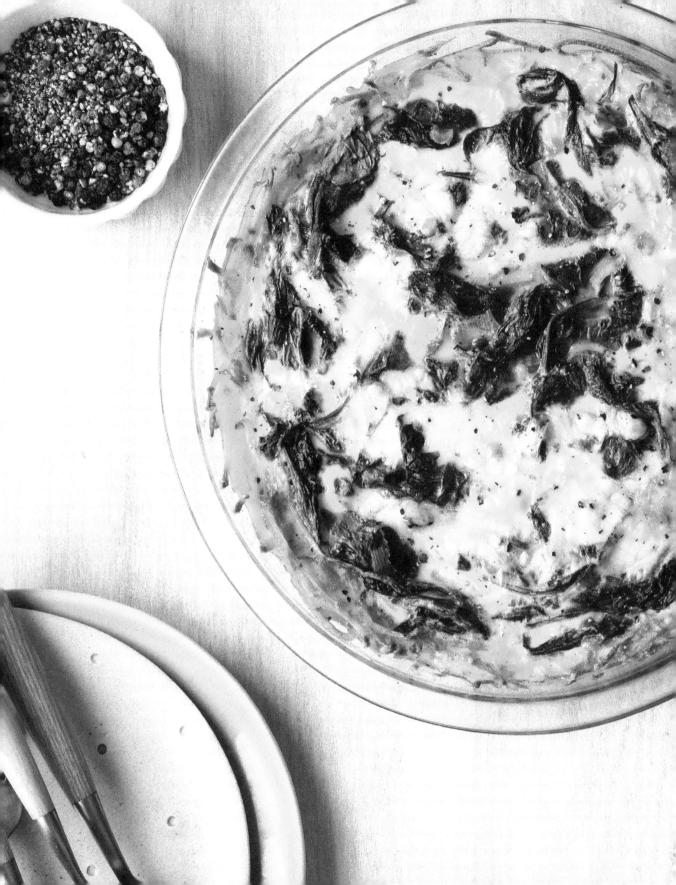

FOUR

Breakfast

Berry-Oat Breakfast Bars

SERVES 12 | **PREP TIME:** 10 minutes | **COOK TIME:** 25 minutes

Rushed early mornings call for a quick yet nutritious breakfast to help power you through the day. This easy recipe is your answer. Loaded with heart-healthy walnuts (feel free to swap in chopped pecans or sliced almonds), seeds, and olive oil, these breakfast bars are healthier and taste better than store-bought bars, and they skip the hard-to-pronounce ingredients. Whip up a batch over the weekend, and you'll be out the door in no time come Monday morning.

2 cups fresh raspberries or blueberries

2 tablespoons sugar

2 tablespoons freshly squeezed lemon juice

1 tablespoon cornstarch

1½ cups rolled oats

½ cup whole-wheat flour

½ cup walnuts

¼ cup chia seeds

¼ cup extra-virgin olive oil

¼ cup honey

1 large egg

1. Preheat the oven to 350° F.

2. In a small saucepan over medium heat, stir together the berries, sugar, lemon juice, and cornstarch. Bring to a simmer. Reduce the heat and simmer for 2 to 3 minutes, until the mixture thickens.

3. In a food processor or high-speed blender, combine the oats, flour, walnuts, and chia seeds. Process until powdered. Add the olive oil, honey, and egg. Pulse a few more times, until well combined. Press half of the mixture into a 9-inch square baking dish.

4. Spread the berry filling over the oat mixture. Add the remaining oat mixture on top of the berries. Bake for 25 minutes, until browned.

5. Let cool completely, cut into 12 pieces, and serve. Store in a covered container for up to 5 days.

PER SERVING: Calories: 201; Total fat: 10g; Saturated fat: 1g; Protein: 5g; Carbs: 26g; Sugar: 9g; Fiber: 5g; Cholesterol: 16mg; Sodium: 8mg

Whole-Grain Breakfast Cookies

MAKES 18 COOKIES | **PREP TIME:** 20 minutes | **COOK TIME:** 10 minutes

Cookies for breakfast with no guilt trip attached? Yes, indeed. These cookies contain no refined sugar—only wholesome, natural sweetness provided by unsweetened applesauce, dried fruit, and coconut. Ground flaxseed is a wonderful addition, being a good source of fiber, magnesium, and several B vitamins. No doubt, these cookies will become a family favorite.

2 cups rolled oats

½ cup whole-wheat flour

¼ cup ground flaxseed

1 teaspoon baking powder

1 cup unsweetened applesauce

2 large eggs

2 tablespoons vegetable oil

2 teaspoons vanilla extract

1 teaspoon ground cinnamon

½ cup dried cherries

¼ cup unsweetened shredded coconut

2 ounces dark chocolate, chopped

1. Preheat the oven to 350° F.

2. In a large bowl, combine the oats, flour, flaxseed, and baking powder. Stir well to mix.

3. In a medium bowl, whisk the applesauce, eggs, vegetable oil, vanilla, and cinnamon. Pour the wet mixture into the dry mixture, and stir until just combined.

4. Fold in the cherries, coconut, and chocolate. Drop tablespoon-size balls of dough onto a baking sheet. Bake for 10 to 12 minutes, until browned and cooked through.

5. Let cool for about 3 minutes, remove from the baking sheet, and cool completely before serving. Store in an airtight container for up to 1 week.

VARIATION TIP: If dried cherries are not your thing, use any other dried fruit you have on hand—raisins, golden raisins, and cranberries all work great.

PER SERVING: Calories: 136; Total fat: 7g; Saturated fat: 3g; Protein: 4g; Carbs: 14g; Sugar: 4g; Fiber: 3g; Cholesterol: 21mg; Sodium: 11mg

Blueberry Breakfast Cake

SERVES 12 | **PREP TIME:** 15 minutes | **COOK TIME:** 45 minutes

Growing up, I remember coffee cake served at breakfast on special occasions. This "cake" is no different, with all its wonderful moist richness, except it's made with healthier whole-wheat pastry and oat flours. If oat flour is something you rarely use, it's easy to make a small batch at home instead of buying it. Simply place the same amount of regular oats in a food processor or high-speed blender, give it a couple of pulses, and voilà—it's done. If using frozen blueberries, no need to thaw. Just avoid overmixing to prevent a purple batter.

FOR THE TOPPING

¼ cup finely chopped walnuts

½ teaspoon ground cinnamon

2 tablespoons butter, chopped into small pieces

2 tablespoons sugar

FOR THE CAKE

Nonstick cooking spray

1 cup whole-wheat pastry flour

1 cup oat flour

¼ cup sugar

2 teaspoons baking powder

1 large egg, beaten

½ cup skim milk

2 tablespoons butter, melted

1 teaspoon grated lemon peel

2 cups fresh or frozen blueberries

TO MAKE THE TOPPING

In a small bowl, stir together the walnuts, cinnamon, butter, and sugar. Set aside.

TO MAKE THE CAKE

1. Preheat the oven to 350° F. Spray a 9-inch square pan with cooking spray. Set aside.

2. In a large bowl, stir together the pastry flour, oat flour, sugar, and baking powder.

3. Add the egg, milk, butter, and lemon peel, and stir until there are no dry spots.

4. Stir in the blueberries, and gently mix until incorporated. Press the batter into the prepared pan, using a spoon to flatten it into the dish.

5. Sprinkle the topping over the cake.

6. Bake for 40 to 45 minutes, until a toothpick inserted into the cake comes out clean, and serve.

TECHNIQUE TIP: This is a thick batter. You will need to press it firmly into the pan, not pour it like cake batter. Use your clean hands or a wooden spoon to press it firmly into the baking dish.

PER SERVING: Calories: 177; Total fat: 7g; Saturated fat: 3g; Protein: 4g; Carbs: 26g; Sugar: 9g; Fiber: 3g; Cholesterol: 26mg; Sodium: 39mg

Whole-Grain Pancakes

SERVES 4 TO 6 | **PREP TIME:** 10 minutes | **COOK TIME:** 15 minutes

Pancakes for breakfast are always a treat, and these are exceptional. Naturally sweetened with honey and made with whole-wheat pastry flour, these pancakes deliver a healthy blend of nutritional goodness. Whole-wheat pastry flour, when compared to white flour, has a lighter yet similar flavor and texture due to its lower protein content.

2 cups whole-wheat pastry flour

4 teaspoons baking powder

2 teaspoons ground cinnamon

½ teaspoon salt

2 cups skim milk, plus more as needed

2 large eggs

1 tablespoon honey

Nonstick cooking spray

Maple syrup, for serving

Fresh fruit, for serving

1. In a large bowl, stir together the flour, baking powder, cinnamon, and salt.

2. Add the milk, eggs, and honey, and stir well to combine. If needed, add more milk, 1 tablespoon at a time, until there are no dry spots and you have a pourable batter.

3. Heat a large skillet over medium-high heat, and spray it with cooking spray.

4. Using a ¼-cup measuring cup, scoop 2 or 3 pancakes into the skillet at a time. Cook for a couple of minutes, until bubbles form on the surface of the pancakes, flip, and cook for 1 to 2 minutes more, until golden brown and cooked through. Repeat with the remaining batter.

5. Serve topped with maple syrup or fresh fruit.

MAKE-AHEAD TIP: Pancakes are easy to make in advance and reheat. If you don't eat them all, transfer to a resealable plastic bag and refrigerate for up to 5 days. Reheat in the toaster or microwave for breakfast in minutes.

PER SERVING: Calories: 392; Total fat: 4g; Saturated fat: 1g; Protein: 15g; Carbs: 71g; Sugar: 11g; Fiber: 9g; Cholesterol: 95mg; Sodium: 396mg

Buckwheat Groats Breakfast Bowl

SERVES 4 | **PREP TIME:** 5 minutes, plus overnight to soak | **COOK TIME:** 10 to 12 minutes

You may be unfamiliar with groats—the hulled kernel of grains—but they are worth a try. Buckwheat is the fruit of a leafy plant with characteristics similar to common cereal grains, but it's actually a seed and gluten free. Packed with vitamins, antioxidants, and protein, it's good for lowering cholesterol and the risk of heart disease. Its nutty flavor is a welcome twist on traditional oatmeal, and with the added pistachios and strawberries, what's not to love?

3 cups skim milk

1 cup buckwheat groats

¼ cup chia seeds

2 teaspoons vanilla extract

½ teaspoon ground cinnamon

Pinch salt

1 cup water

½ cup unsalted pistachios

2 cups sliced fresh strawberries

¼ cup cacao nibs (optional)

1. In a large bowl, stir together the milk, groats, chia seeds, vanilla, cinnamon, and salt. Cover and refrigerate overnight.

2. The next morning, transfer the soaked mixture to a medium pot and add the water. Bring to a boil over medium-high heat, reduce the heat to maintain a simmer, and cook for 10 to 12 minutes, until the buckwheat is tender and thickened.

3. Transfer to bowls and serve, topped with the pistachios, strawberries, and cacao nibs (if using).

INGREDIENT TIP: Buckwheat groats are not the same thing as kasha, which can be a variety of different cereal grains. Buckwheat groats are fruit seeds resembling a small lentil or split pea. Look for them in health food stores, bulk food sections, or online.

PER SERVING: Calories: 340; Total fat: 8g; Saturated fat: 1g; Protein: 15g; Carbs: 52g; Sugar: 14g; Fiber: 10g; Cholesterol: 4mg; Sodium: 140mg

Peach Muesli Bake

SERVES 8 | **PREP TIME:** 10 minutes | **COOK TIME:** 40 minutes

I'm a big fan of all things muesli. Popular around the world, muesli is a tasty mix of fruit, nuts, seeds, and grains served warm or cold. A nutritional winner, muesli tends to have less sugar and fewer calories than other cereals at the grocery store. Add your favorite nut, and substitute berries for the peaches if you like. Either way, this recipe is loaded with protein, fiber, and vitamins C and E. Serve with plain nonfat Greek yogurt for a nutritious and tasty breakfast.

Nonstick cooking spray

2 cups skim milk

1½ cups rolled oats

½ cup chopped walnuts

1 large egg

2 tablespoons maple syrup

1 teaspoon ground cinnamon

1 teaspoon baking powder

½ teaspoon salt

2 to 3 peaches, sliced

1. Preheat the oven to 375° F. Spray a 9-inch square baking dish with cooking spray. Set aside.

2. In a large bowl, stir together the milk, oats, walnuts, egg, maple syrup, cinnamon, baking powder, and salt. Spread half the mixture in the prepared baking dish.

3. Place half the peaches in a single layer across the oat mixture.

4. Spread the remaining oat mixture over the top. Add the remaining peaches in a thin layer over the oats. Bake for 35 to 40 minutes, uncovered, until thickened and browned.

5. Cut into 8 squares and serve warm.

INGREDIENT TIP: While oats are inherently gluten free, unless they are labeled as such, it is likely they have been contaminated with gluten during processing. Be sure to check the labels if you are gluten sensitive.

PER SERVING: Calories: 138; Total fat: 3g; Saturated fat: 1g; Protein: 6g; Carbs: 22g; Sugar: 10g; Fiber: 3g; Cholesterol: 24mg; Sodium: 191mg

Steel-Cut Oatmeal Bowl with Fruit and Nuts

SERVES 4 | **PREP TIME:** 5 minutes | **COOK TIME:** 20 minutes

Here's the only steel-cut oatmeal recipe you'll ever need—it's foolproof, and the nutty, chewy texture will leave you happily satisfied and ready to face the day. Topped with heart-healthy nuts and fresh fruit, it's a perfect building block for an ultra-nutritious breakfast. Test your adventurous side by spicing things up with added nutmeg, cloves, or ginger. You can also cut cooking time in half by soaking the oats the night before.

1 cup steel-cut oats

2 cups almond milk

¾ cup water

1 teaspoon ground cinnamon

¼ teaspoon salt

2 cups chopped fresh fruit, such as blueberries, strawberries, raspberries, or peaches

½ cup chopped walnuts

¼ cup chia seeds

1. In a medium saucepan over medium-high heat, combine the oats, almond milk, water, cinnamon, and salt. Bring to a boil, reduce the heat to low, and simmer for 15 to 20 minutes, until the oats are softened and thickened.

2. Top each bowl with ½ cup of fresh fruit, 2 tablespoons of walnuts, and 1 tablespoon of chia seeds before serving.

MAKE-AHEAD TIP: One of the best things about steel-cut oats is they taste great when reheated. Make this up to 3 days in advance and reheat in the microwave or on the stovetop for a quick breakfast. Add a little extra almond milk when serving to loosen the oats up, if desired.

PER SERVING: Calories: 288; Total fat: 11g; Saturated fat: 1g; Protein: 10g; Carbs: 38g; Sugar: 7g; Fiber: 10g; Cholesterol: 0mg; Sodium: 329mg

Whole-Grain Dutch Baby Pancake

SERVES 4 | **PREP TIME:** 5 minutes | **COOK TIME:** 25 minutes

This isn't your usual way of making pancakes—it's even easier. Just blend the ingredients, pour the batter into an oven-safe skillet, and bake while you prep fresh fruit as a side. The whole-wheat flour boosts the fiber content and adds a nutty flavor. As it bakes, the pancake will rise and then fall when brought out of the oven. A dusting of powdered sugar tops it off when you're ready to indulge.

2 tablespoons coconut oil

½ cup whole-wheat flour

¼ cup skim milk

3 large eggs

1 teaspoon vanilla extract

½ teaspoon baking powder

¼ teaspoon salt

¼ teaspoon ground cinnamon

Powdered sugar, for dusting

1. Preheat the oven to 400° F.

2. Put the coconut oil in a medium oven-safe skillet, and place the skillet in the oven to melt the oil while it preheats.

3. In a blender, combine the flour, milk, eggs, vanilla, baking powder, salt, and cinnamon. Process until smooth.

4. Carefully remove the skillet from the oven and tilt to spread the oil around evenly.

5. Pour the batter into the skillet and return it to the oven for 23 to 25 minutes, until the pancake puffs and lightly browns.

6. Remove, dust lightly with powdered sugar, cut into 4 wedges, and serve.

PER SERVING: Calories: 195; Total fat: 11g; Saturated fat: 7g; Protein: 8g; Carbs: 16g; Sugar: 1g; Fiber: 2g; Cholesterol: 140mg; Sodium: 209mg

Mushroom, Zucchini, and Onion Frittata

SERVES 4 | **PREP TIME:** 10 minutes | **COOK TIME:** 20 minutes

This lovely breakfast frittata also makes a perfect brunch. It's prepared with minimal dishes so cleanup is quick (my favorite kind of recipe!). *Frittata* is an Italian word for omelet, and it is usually baked in the oven. No worries if zucchini isn't your favorite veggie. Throw in any veggies you like to make it your own. Consider adding fresh herbs, such as rosemary, which pairs nicely with the mushrooms, eggs, and onion.

1 tablespoon extra-virgin olive oil

½ onion, chopped

1 medium zucchini, chopped

1½ cups sliced mushrooms

6 large eggs, beaten

2 tablespoons skim milk

Salt

Freshly ground black pepper

1 ounce feta cheese, crumbled

1. Preheat the oven to 400° F.

2. In a medium oven-safe skillet over medium-high heat, heat the olive oil.

3. Add the onion, and sauté for 3 to 5 minutes, until translucent.

4. Add the zucchini and mushrooms, and cook for 3 to 5 more minutes, until the vegetables are tender.

5. Meanwhile, in a small bowl, whisk the eggs, milk, salt, and pepper. Pour the mixture into the skillet, stirring to combine, and transfer the skillet to the oven. Cook for 7 to 9 minutes, until set.

6. Sprinkle with the feta cheese, and cook for 1 to 2 minutes more, until heated through.

7. Remove, cut into 4 wedges, and serve.

MAKE-AHEAD TIP: The vegetables for this dish can be chopped 1 to 2 days in advance, making it even quicker in the morning when preparing breakfast. Once cooked, you can refrigerate the frittata wedges in a covered container for 3 to 4 days.

PER SERVING: Calories: 178; Total fat: 13g; Saturated fat: 4g; Protein: 12g; Carbs: 5g; Sugar: 3g; Fiber: 1g; Cholesterol: 285mg; Sodium: 234mg

Spinach and Cheese Quiche

SERVES 4 TO 6 | **PREP TIME:** 10 minutes, plus 10 minutes to rest | **COOK TIME:** 50 minutes

Everyone will come bounding out of bed when you make this mouthwatering Spinach and Cheese Quiche. Not your run-of-the-mill quiche, this recipe uses a potato crust as a shell, which provides a delightful, homespun touch. Leave the potatoes unpeeled—the skins add extra fiber and give it a rustic, hearty look. Round out the meal with freshly sliced oranges or strawberries for a vitamin C and antioxidant boost.

Nonstick cooking spray

8 ounces Yukon Gold potatoes, shredded

1 tablespoon plus 2 teaspoons extra-virgin olive oil, divided

1 teaspoon salt, divided

Freshly ground black pepper

1 onion, finely chopped

1 (10-ounce) bag fresh spinach

4 large eggs

½ cup skim milk

1 ounce Gruyère cheese, shredded

1. Preheat the oven to 350° F. Spray a 9-inch pie dish with cooking spray. Set aside.

2. In a small bowl, toss the potatoes with 2 teaspoons of olive oil, ½ teaspoon of salt, and season with pepper. Press the potatoes into the bottom and sides of the pie dish to form a thin, even layer. Bake for 20 minutes, until golden brown. Remove from the oven and set aside to cool.

3. In a large skillet over medium-high heat, heat the remaining 1 tablespoon of olive oil.

4. Add the onion, and sauté for 3 to 5 minutes, until softened.

5. By handfuls, add the spinach, stirring between each addition, until it just starts to wilt before adding more. Cook for about 1 minute, until it cooks down.

6. In a medium bowl, whisk the eggs and milk. Add the Gruyère, and season with the remaining ½ teaspoon of salt and some pepper. Fold the eggs into the spinach. Pour the mixture into the pie dish and bake for 25 minutes, until the eggs are set.

7. Let rest for 10 minutes before serving.

PER SERVING: Calories: 445; Total fat: 14g; Saturated fat: 4g; Protein: 19g; Carbs: 68g; Sugar: 6g; Fiber: 7g; Cholesterol: 193mg; Sodium: 773mg

Egg and Veggie Breakfast Cups

SERVES 8 | **PREP TIME:** 10 minutes | **COOK TIME:** 25 minutes

Start your day with a good source of colorful antioxidant-rich veggies! The protein-rich eggs and fiber-filled veggies also help slow digestion, leaving you feeling fuller longer. Prep the veggies the night before to make this recipe a snap the next morning. Baking these individual cups in a muffin tin aids portion control, and any leftovers can be refrigerated to keep handy for quick meals to enjoy over several days.

Nonstick cooking spray

1 tablespoon extra-virgin olive oil

1 onion, finely chopped

½ green bell pepper, finely chopped

½ red bell pepper, finely chopped

2 garlic cloves, minced

8 large eggs

Salt

Freshly ground black pepper

¼ cup sun-dried tomatoes, finely chopped (see tip)

1. Preheat the oven to 350° F. Spray 8 wells of a muffin tin with cooking spray. Set aside.

2. In a small skillet over medium heat, heat the olive oil.

3. Add the onion and green and red bell peppers, and sauté for 4 to 5 minutes, until they begin to soften. Add the garlic and cook for 30 seconds more, until fragrant. Remove from the heat.

4. In a large bowl, whisk the eggs and season with salt and pepper. Stir in the vegetable mixture and the sun-dried tomatoes. Divide the egg mixture among the 8 prepared muffin cups. Bake for 16 to 20 minutes, until the eggs are set.

5. Remove and serve. Refrigerate leftovers in a covered container for up to 5 days.

INGREDIENT TIP: Use oil-packed or dried sun-dried tomatoes, but be sure to reconstitute the dried tomatoes before you begin. To reconstitute, in a small bowl, combine a scant ¼ cup tomatoes with 1 cup water and ¼ teaspoon salt. Cover and microwave on high for 2 minutes. Let rest for 5 minutes, still covered, until tender. Drain, if needed, and finely chop.

PER SERVING: Calories: 102; Total fat: 7g; Saturated fat: 2g; Protein: 7g; Carbs: 4g; Sugar: 2g; Fiber: 1g; Cholesterol: 186mg; Sodium: 126mg

Breakfast Tostada

SERVES 4 | **PREP TIME:** 5 minutes | **COOK TIME:** 20 minutes

Here is healthy made easy. This Breakfast Tostada comes together in minutes and is powerfully nutritious, thanks to the refried beans and avocado. Canned refried beans are a rich source of protein and magnesium and provide both soluble and insoluble fiber, which is good for fighting heart disease. Avocado, a fruit, contains more potassium than bananas and is loaded with heart-healthy monounsaturated fat, helping reduce cholesterol and triglyceride levels.

Nonstick cooking spray

4 corn tortillas

½ cup fat-free refried beans

1 tablespoon extra-virgin olive oil

4 large eggs

Salt

Freshly ground black pepper

1 avocado, peeled, pitted, and sliced

½ cup salsa

¼ cup crumbled feta cheese

1. Preheat the oven to 350° F. Spray a baking sheet with nonstick cooking spray.

2. Place the tortillas on the prepared baking sheet, overlapping the edges if needed. Bake for 12 to 15 minutes until crisp. Remove from the oven and set aside.

3. In a small pot over medium heat, warm the refried beans.

4. In a small skillet over medium-high heat, heat the olive oil.

5. Crack the eggs into the skillet. Fry for 3 to 5 minutes, depending on preferred doneness. Season lightly with salt and pepper.

6. Assemble the tostadas by spreading a layer of beans on each tortilla, topping each with 1 egg, a couple of avocado slices, 2 tablespoons of salsa, and 1 tablespoon of feta cheese.

MAKE-AHEAD TIP: Bake the tortillas the night before and assemble the tostadas in the morning.

PER SERVING: Calories: 290; Total fat: 18g; Saturated fat: 5g; Protein: 12g; Carbs: 23g; Sugar: 2g; Fiber: 7g; Cholesterol: 194mg; Sodium: 549mg

Egg and Potato Scramble

SERVES 4 | **PREP TIME:** 10 minutes | **COOK TIME:** 25 minutes

Scrambled eggs for breakfast are always a good choice, and when potatoes are added, it's even better. Full of flavor and easy to assemble, this one-skillet dish will get your morning started right. Starting with the potatoes allows them to form a nice crispiness on the edges. This recipe lends itself to improvisation: Throw in other nonstarchy veggies, such as chopped tomatoes, mushrooms, spinach, or baby kale.

1 tablespoon extra-virgin olive oil

2 cups chopped (½-inch pieces) potatoes

1 onion, finely chopped

½ green bell pepper, finely chopped

6 large eggs

½ teaspoon salt

¼ teaspoon freshly ground black pepper

2 tablespoons chopped fresh parsley

1. In a large skillet or wok over medium heat, heat the olive oil.

2. Add the potatoes. Cook for 12 to 15 minutes, stirring occasionally, until browned and nearly fork-tender.

3. Add the onion and green bell pepper. Continue to cook for 3 to 5 minutes more, until the vegetables begin to soften.

4. In a medium bowl, whisk the eggs and season with the salt and pepper. Pour the eggs into the potatoes and cook for 3 to 4 minutes, stirring regularly, until set.

5. Serve sprinkled with the parsley.

MAKE-AHEAD TIP: Cook the potatoes and onions the night before to make this breakfast come together in minutes. After completing step 3, let the vegetables cool, transfer to an airtight container, and refrigerate until needed.

PER SERVING: Calories: 180; Total fat: 11g; Saturated fat: 3g; Protein: 11g; Carbs: 10g; Sugar: 3g; Fiber: 2g; Cholesterol: 279mg; Sodium: 401mg

Sweet Potato Hash with Eggs

SERVES 4 | **PREP TIME:** 10 minutes | **COOK TIME:** 25 minutes

This grain-free recipe serves up sweet potatoes, an excellent source of vitamin A, and prosciutto, a thinly sliced Italian ham that adds incredible flavor even in small amounts. It takes little time to assemble, and any leftovers can be reheated; just wait to fry the eggs until right before serving.

2 tablespoons extra-virgin olive oil

½ onion, chopped

2 medium sweet potatoes, chopped into ½-inch pieces

2 slices prosciutto, cut into thin strips

4 large eggs

¼ teaspoon salt

Freshly ground black pepper

2 tablespoons chopped fresh parsley

1. In a large skillet over medium-high heat, heat the olive oil.

2. Add the onion, and sauté for about 2 minutes, until just beginning to soften.

3. Add the sweet potatoes, and sauté for 12 to 15 minutes, stirring occasionally, until the sweet potatoes are fork-tender and browned.

4. Stir in the prosciutto and cook for 1 minute more, until heated through. Once the sweet potatoes are cooked, push them to the side of the skillet.

5. Crack the eggs into the skillet and cook for 3 to 5 minutes, until set. Season with the salt and some pepper.

6. Serve the hash topped by one egg per serving, garnished with the parsley.

PER SERVING: Calories: 228; Total fat: 13g; Saturated fat: 3g; Protein: 13g; Carbs: 15g; Sugar: 4g; Fiber: 2g; Cholesterol: 199mg; Sodium: 616mg

Chicken Chilaquiles with Eggs

SERVES 4 | **PREP TIME:** 10 minutes | **COOK TIME:** 45 minutes

Chilaquiles are a traditional Mexican dish consisting of fried tortilla strips topped with a spicy sauce and cheese. Often served for breakfast or brunch, they're delicious any time of day. Here, I use baked corn tortillas instead of calorie-laden fried tortilla strips. This dish is an excellent way to use up leftover cooked chicken, and is a great make-ahead meal that stores and reheats nicely; just wait to cook the egg until after the casserole is reheated.

Nonstick cooking spray

4 corn tortillas

2 tablespoons extra-virgin olive oil

½ onion, chopped

1 (15-ounce) can no-salt-added diced tomatoes

1 canned chipotle chile in adobo, chopped

1 teaspoon adobo sauce (from the can)

2 cups chopped fresh spinach

1 cup cooked shredded chicken

½ cup shredded Monterey Jack cheese

4 large eggs

Chopped scallion, white and green parts, for garnishing

1. Preheat the oven to 350° F. Spray a 9-by-13-inch baking dish with cooking spray.

2. Place the tortillas in the prepared baking dish in a single layer, overlapping the edges as needed. Bake for 12 to 15 minutes, until the tortillas harden and begin to lightly brown. Remove from the oven.

3. Meanwhile, in a large skillet over medium-high heat, heat the olive oil.

4. Add the onion, and sauté for 3 to 5 minutes, until softened.

5. Stir in the tomatoes, chile in adobo, and adobo sauce. Cook for 5 to 6 minutes, until the oil begins to separate.

6. Add the spinach, and stir until wilted. Remove from the heat.

7. Remove the tortillas from the baking dish, and set aside. Spread about ½ cup of the tomato mixture across the bottom of the dish. Place the tortillas back in the dish. Top each with ¼ cup of chicken, ¼ cup of tomato sauce, and 2 tablespoons of cheese.

8. Cover the dish with aluminum foil and bake for 20 to 25 minutes, until the cheese melts and the casserole is bubbling.

9. Remove the foil, and use a spoon to make 4 indents in the casserole. Crack the eggs into the indents, taking care not to break the yolks.

10. Return the dish to the oven and bake for 3 to 7 minutes more, depending on how firm you like your eggs.

11. Serve garnished with the scallion.

INGREDIENT TIP: Chipotle chiles in adobo sauce are commonly found in the Mexican food section of many grocery stores. While the cans are typically small, you will have several leftover chiles after making this recipe. Refrigerate them for up to 1 month, or freeze for up to 1 year and use to heat up many dishes with their smoky flavor.

PER SERVING: Calories: 319; Total fat: 19g; Saturated fat: 6g; Protein: 23g; Carbs: 17g; Sugar: 4g; Fiber: 3g; Cholesterol: 227mg; Sodium: 320mg

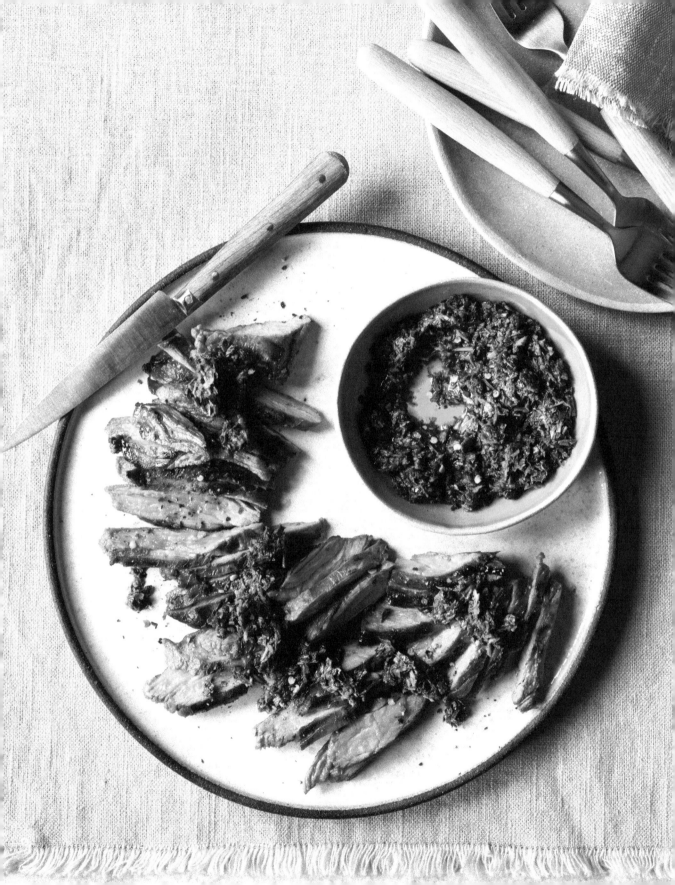

— FIVE —

Mains

◄ FLANK STEAK WITH CHIMICHURRI, PAGE 96

Margherita Pizza

SERVES 6 | **PREP TIME:** 15 minutes, plus 1 hour 15 minutes to rest | **COOK TIME:** 20 minutes

Margherita Pizza—supposedly named after Margherita of Savoy, onetime queen consort of Italy—is a favorite of mine, and you'll love it, too. This Neapolitan pizza is made with tomato, sliced mozzarella, basil, and extra-virgin olive oil; it's vegetarian, and skipping any meat toppings makes it much lower in fat. In addition, the crust is made using part whole-wheat flour. Add a side salad loaded with veggies and your meal is ready. No matter how you slice it, pizza Margherita is delicious.

FOR THE DOUGH

1 cup warm water (about 110°F)

1 teaspoon sugar

2¼ teaspoons active dry yeast (1 [¼-ounce] package)

1½ cups whole-wheat flour

1½ cups all-purpose flour

2 tablespoons extra-virgin olive oil, divided

1 teaspoon salt

FOR THE PIZZA

Extra-virgin olive oil, for preparing the baking sheet

1 (14-ounce) can no-salt-added diced tomatoes, drained

8 ounces mozzarella cheese, sliced

¼ cup fresh basil leaves

TO MAKE THE DOUGH

1. In a stand mixer fitted with a dough hook, combine the warm water, sugar, and yeast. Mix well and let sit for about 5 minutes, until bubbly.

2. Add the whole-wheat and all-purpose flours, 1 tablespoon of olive oil, and the salt. Mix on low speed until the dough comes together. Increase the speed to medium and continue mixing for about 5 minutes, until the dough becomes elastic and shiny.

3. Coat a large bowl with the remaining 1 tablespoon of olive oil, and transfer the dough to the bowl. Cover the bowl with plastic wrap, set it in a warm place, and let rise until doubled in size, about 1 hour.

4. Punch the dough down, and form it into a ball. Let rest for 15 minutes.

1. Preheat the oven to 500° F. Lightly coat a baking sheet with olive oil.

2. In a blender, process the tomatoes until puréed.

3. Place the dough ball on the prepared baking sheet, and use your hands to stretch and shape it to the size of the baking sheet.

4. Spread the tomato sauce on the pizza dough. Cover with the mozzarella slices, and top with the basil leaves. Bake for 12 to 18 minutes, until the cheese is melted and the crust is browned in spots.

5. Remove from the oven and let cool for 5 minutes. Cut into 6 slices and serve.

MAKE-AHEAD TIP: The dough can be made up to 2 days in advance and refrigerated at step 3 after covering it with plastic wrap but before letting it rise. Bring the dough to room temperature before continuing with the recipe.

PER SERVING: Calories: 426; Total fat: 13g; Saturated fat: 5g; Protein: 21g; Carbs: 60g; Sugar: 3g; Fiber: 6g; Cholesterol: 20mg; Sodium: 620mg

Chickpea, Tomato, and Kale Soup

SERVES 4 | **PREP TIME:** 10 minutes | **COOK TIME:** 15 minutes

Nothing sounds quite so good on a brisk day as a delicious bowl of hot soup. Using ingredients that come together easily, this hearty soup overflows with fiber, vitamins A and C, and potassium. Be sure to use low-sodium varieties when buying canned goods. This soup is perfect for a quick dinner solution—just 10 minutes of prep and 15 minutes to cook. Served with a crusty loaf of bread, it's a nourishing crowd-pleaser.

1 tablespoon extra-virgin olive oil

1 onion, chopped

3 garlic cloves, minced

1 (15.5-ounce) can chickpeas, drained

1 (15-ounce) can no-salt-added diced tomatoes

4 cups low-sodium vegetable broth

4 cups finely chopped kale leaves

½ teaspoon salt

Freshly ground black pepper

1 ounce Parmesan cheese, shredded

1. In a large pot over medium-high heat, heat the olive oil.

2. Add the onion, and sauté for 3 to 5 minutes, until softened.

3. Add the garlic, and cook for 30 seconds, until fragrant.

4. Stir in the chickpeas and tomatoes and their juices. Add the vegetable broth, and bring to a boil. Reduce the heat to low, add the kale, and simmer for 2 to 3 minutes, until the kale wilts. Season with the salt and some pepper.

5. Serve topped with the Parmesan.

INGREDIENT TIP: Save time on chopping by purchasing a bag of prechopped kale. Alternatively, baby kale leaves are also a quick option that requires no prep work. The tender leaves cook more quickly than mature ones, so cut the simmer time to 1 minute.

PER SERVING: Calories: 273; Total fat: 6g; Saturated fat: 2g; Protein: 13g; Carbs: 42g; Sugar: 3g; Fiber: 7g; Cholesterol: 5mg; Sodium: 823mg

Lentil and Vegetable Soup

SERVES 6 | **PREP TIME:** 10 minutes | **COOK TIME:** 30 minutes

Lentils are one of the most versatile and nutritious foods for regulating blood sugar. Low in fat, cholesterol free, high in folate, potassium, and iron, and a rich source of fiber, lentils have it all. Combined with vegetables, it's a nutritional match made in heaven. Best of all, unlike other beans, lentils require no presoaking, making them perfect for a weeknight meal. Make life simple and healthier—start eating lentils today!

2 tablespoons extra-virgin olive oil

2 carrots, chopped

2 celery stalks, chopped

1 onion, chopped

3 garlic cloves, minced

2 cups dried brown lentils, rinsed

4 cups low-sodium vegetable broth

1 cup water

4 cups chopped fresh spinach

½ teaspoon salt

¼ teaspoon freshly ground black pepper

1. In a large pot over medium heat, heat the olive oil.

2. Add the carrots, celery, and onion, and sauté for 3 to 5 minutes, until the onion is softened.

3. Add the garlic. Cook, stirring, for about 30 seconds, until fragrant.

4. Add the lentils, vegetable broth, and water, and bring to a boil. Reduce the heat to maintain a simmer, cover the pot, and cook for 20 minutes, until the lentils are tender.

5. Turn off the heat, and stir in the spinach. Let heat for 1 to 2 minutes, until wilted.

6. Season with the salt and pepper and serve.

VARIATION TIP: Vegetable broth gives this soup a lovely flavor, while keeping it vegetarian. However, feel free to use chicken broth or even water to make this soup. If you do use water, add a bit more salt and be sure to taste it before serving.

PER SERVING: Calories: 274; Total fat: 6g; Saturated fat: 1g; Protein: 17g; Carbs: 39g; Sugar: 2g; Fiber: 8g; Cholesterol: 0mg; Sodium: 276mg

Black Bean Soup

SERVES 4 | **PREP TIME:** 5 minutes | **COOK TIME:** 20 minutes

Talk about a flavorful soup. Simple to put together and ready in less than 30 minutes, this is a recipe you'll come back to often. Black beans are a powerhouse of protein, fiber, magnesium, potassium, and vitamin K, and this recipe makes one of the most satisfying, hearty soups—good any time of year. Throw in some frozen corn or fire-roasted tomatoes to ramp up the flavor, if you like. Pair it with a dark leafy green salad and you've got a meal to feel good about.

2 tablespoons extra-virgin olive oil

1 onion, chopped

3 garlic cloves, minced

2 (15-ounce) cans black beans, rinsed and drained

3 cups low-sodium vegetable broth

1 teaspoon ground cumin

½ teaspoon salt

Crumbled feta cheese, for serving

1. In a large pot over medium-high heat, heat the olive oil.

2. Add the onion, and sauté for 3 to 5 minutes, until softened.

3. Add the garlic, and cook for 30 seconds more, until fragrant.

4. Stir in the black beans, vegetable broth, cumin, and salt. Bring to a boil, reduce the heat to maintain a simmer, and cook for 10 minutes, until slightly thickened and the flavors meld.

5. Using a potato masher, mash about half the beans in the soup. Serve, topped with feta cheese.

MAKE-AHEAD TIP: Soups tend to get better with age as the flavors meld. This soup will keep well for about 4 days in the refrigerator, so make it early in the week and enjoy it when you need a quick meal.

PER SERVING: Calories: 333; Total fat: 10g; Saturated fat: 2g; Protein: 18g; Carbs: 45g; Sugar: 2g; Fiber: 16g; Cholesterol: 6mg; Sodium: 426mg

Falafel Sandwich

SERVES 6 | **PREP TIME:** 15 minutes | **COOK TIME:** 15 minutes

Falafel is one of the most delicious ways to get more chickpeas on the menu. Nestled in pita bread (use whole-wheat bread for added nutrition), these Middle Eastern chickpea patties, seasoned with onion and spices, make a filling legume-based meal. You can also skip the pitas, serving the falafel on a bed of lightly seasoned greens.

2 (15-ounce) cans chickpeas, drained

1 medium onion, roughly chopped

5 garlic cloves, minced, divided

¼ cup packed fresh parsley leaves

Juice of 1 lemon

2 tablespoons extra-virgin olive oil, divided

1 teaspoon ground cumin

1 teaspoon ground coriander

1¼ teaspoons salt, divided

2 teaspoons baking powder

½ cup plain nonfat Greek yogurt

3 whole-wheat pita pockets, halved

Sliced cucumbers, for serving

Sliced tomatoes, for serving

1. In a food processor, combine the chickpeas, onion, 3 garlic cloves, parsley, lemon juice, 1 tablespoon of olive oil, cumin, coriander, and 1 teaspoon of salt. Pulse several times, until the chickpeas and onions are chopped coarsely and mixed but not puréed. Add the baking powder and pulse several more times, until it is mixed in and the mixture forms into a ball. Form the mixture into 12 small balls, and press the balls into patties.

2. In a small bowl, whisk the yogurt with the remaining ¼ teaspoon of salt and 2 garlic cloves. Set aside.

3. In a large skillet over medium heat, heat the remaining 1 tablespoon of olive oil.

4. Working in batches, cook the patties for 2 to 3 minutes per side, gently flipping once during cooking, until browned and crisp.

5. To serve, place two patties into a half pita, top with cucumber and tomato slices, and garnish with a spoonful of yogurt.

PER SERVING: Calories: 356; Total fat: 8g; Saturated fat: 1g; Protein: 13g; Carbs: 61g; Sugar: 4g; Fiber: 11g; Cholesterol: 1mg; Sodium: 1,154mg

Vegetable Chowder

SERVES 8 | **PREP TIME:** 20 minutes | **COOK TIME:** 25 minutes

Packed with antioxidants and fiber-rich veggies, this Vegetable Chowder is not your typical cream soup. While it does have the same luxurious taste, the cream is replaced by skim milk and sharp Cheddar for a rich, delicious flavor. Unfamiliar with jicama? This tasty, nutrient-dense tuber (native to Mexico) has a mild flavor and satisfying crunch. Make this soup on a weekend, and you'll be covered for several meals during the week ahead.

1 tablespoon extra-virgin olive oil

3 large carrots, chopped

3 celery stalks, chopped

1 large onion, chopped

3 garlic cloves, minced

1 (32-ounce) carton low-sodium vegetable broth

2 russet potatoes, peeled and chopped into ½-inch cubes

1 small jicama, peeled and chopped into ½-inch cubes

1 teaspoon salt

½ teaspoon dried thyme

½ teaspoon freshly ground black pepper

Pinch ground cayenne pepper (optional)

2 medium broccoli crowns, cut into small florets

1 small cauliflower, cut into small florets

4 tablespoons butter

6 tablespoons whole-wheat flour

3 cups skim milk

1 cup shredded sharp Cheddar cheese

1. In a large pot over medium-high heat, heat the olive oil.

2. Add the carrots, celery, and onion, and sauté for 3 to 5 minutes, until the onion begins to soften and brown.

3. Add the garlic, and sauté for 30 seconds, until fragrant.

4. Pour in the vegetable broth, and add the potatoes, jicama, salt, thyme, pepper, and cayenne (if using). Bring to a boil, reduce the heat to medium, and simmer for 10 to 12 minutes, until the potatoes are nearly done.

5. Add the broccoli and cauliflower, and continue cooking for 5 to 7 more minutes, until the vegetables are tender.

6. Meanwhile, in a medium pot over medium heat, melt the butter.

7. Stir in the flour, and cook for about 1 minute, stirring constantly.

8. Adding a small amount at a time, whisk in the milk until smooth. Pour the milk mixture into the soup, and stir to combine.

9. Add the cheese, stir until melted, and serve.

MAKE-AHEAD TIP: This soup reheats wonderfully and is perfect to make ahead. Prepare up to 3 to 4 days in advance and heat on the stove or in the microwave for a quick, nourishing meal.

PER SERVING: Calories: 257; Total fat: 13g; Saturated fat: 7g; Protein: 12g; Carbs: 32g; Sugar: 10g; Fiber: 8g; Cholesterol: 32mg; Sodium: 556mg

Butternut Squash and Mushroom Lasagna

SERVES 8 | **PREP TIME:** 20 minutes, plus 10 minutes to stand | **COOK TIME:** 55 minutes

Vegetarian lasagna never tasted so good. Layers of noodles (to shorten cooking time, use the no-boil kind), squash, fresh mushrooms, and low-fat cottage and ricotta cheeses combine for a wonderful dish that will leave you feeling warm and satisfied. This meatless meal gets a hearty flavor boost from the mushrooms, while fresh herbs provide a nice flavor punch. Freeze leftovers for a fantastic no-prep meal down the road on a busier day.

1 (2-pound) butternut squash

2 tablespoons butter

1 onion, chopped

8 ounces brown mushrooms, chopped

Salt

Freshly ground black pepper

1 (15-ounce) container low-fat ricotta cheese

1 (15-ounce) container low-fat cottage cheese

2 large eggs

3 tablespoons chopped fresh thyme, divided

3 tablespoons chopped fresh sage, divided

1½ cups grated mozzarella cheese

½ cup grated Parmesan cheese

1 (9-ounce) package no-boil lasagna noodles

1. Poke the squash several times with a fork. Microwave it at high power for 6 to 8 minutes, depending on your microwave, until tender. Set aside and let cool.

2. Preheat the oven to 350°F.

3. Meanwhile, in a large skillet over medium-high heat, melt the butter.

4. Add the onion, and cook for 3 to 5 minutes, until just starting to soften.

5. Add the mushrooms, and cook until the liquid evaporates, about 5 minutes. Season lightly with salt and pepper.

6. In a large bowl, stir together the ricotta, cottage cheese, eggs, and 1½ tablespoons each of thyme and sage until well mixed.

7. Using a vegetable peeler or sharp knife, peel the squash and chop into ½-inch pieces. Transfer to another large bowl, and gently toss with the remaining 1½ tablespoons each of sage and thyme.

8. Spread about 1 cup of the ricotta cheese mixture on the bottom of a 9-by-13-inch baking dish.

9. Arrange 3 noodles on top of the cheese. On the noodles, spread about 1 cup of the ricotta mixture, 1 cup of squash, ½ cup of mushrooms, and ½ cup of mozzarella cheese.

10. Add 3 more noodles, and repeat the same process for another layer.

11. Top with the remaining 3 noodles, the remaining 1 cup of ricotta mixture, and the remaining ½ cup of mozzarella. Sprinkle the top with the grated Parmesan cheese. Cover the dish with aluminum foil and bake for 40 minutes, until the noodles are softened and the lasagna is bubbly.

12. Remove the foil and bake for 5 minutes more, until the top is golden brown.

13. Let stand for 10 minutes before serving.

PER SERVING: Calories: 352; Total fat: 15g; Saturated fat: 9g; Protein: 26g; Carbs: 30g; Sugar: 4g; Fiber: 3g; Cholesterol: 104mg; Sodium: 545mg

Spaghetti with Chickpea and Mushroom Marinara

SERVES 4 | **PREP TIME:** 15 minutes | **COOK TIME:** 25 minutes

Looking for a vegetarian spaghetti option? Here's your answer—and a whole new pleasing way of serving a healthy, low-fat meal. This dish is packed with protein-rich chickpeas, but it's the mushrooms that provide a meaty flavor. Be sure to use whole-wheat pasta, and be mindful of the portion size to reduce carbohydrate intake.

1 (15-ounce) can low-sodium chickpeas, rinsed and drained

1 tablespoon extra-virgin olive oil

8 ounces fresh mushrooms, finely chopped

1 onion, finely chopped

3 garlic cloves, minced

1 (28-ounce) can no-salt-added whole tomatoes

1 tablespoon honey

½ teaspoon salt

¼ teaspoon red pepper flakes

Freshly ground black pepper

8 ounces whole-wheat spaghetti

1. In a food processor, pulse the chickpeas several times until coarsely ground.

2. In a large skillet over medium-high heat, heat the olive oil.

3. Add the mushrooms and onion, and cook for 5 to 7 minutes, until softened and the liquid has evaporated.

4. Add the garlic, and cook for 30 seconds, until fragrant.

5. Use your hand or a spoon to break apart the tomatoes in the can. Add the tomatoes and their juices to the skillet, along with the honey, salt, red pepper flakes, and black pepper. Add the chickpeas to the skillet. Bring to a boil, reduce the heat to medium-low, and simmer for 10 minutes.

6. Meanwhile, fill a large pot halfway with water and bring to a boil over high heat. Cook the pasta according to the package directions, until al dente. Drain.

7. Serve the pasta topped with the marinara sauce.

MAKE-AHEAD TIP: Make the sauce and noodles up to 3 days in advance. Refrigerate in separate containers until ready to serve, then stir together and heat on the stovetop or in the microwave.

PER SERVING: Calories: 456; Total fat: 6g; Saturated fat: 1g; Protein: 18g; Carbs: 88g; Sugar: 12g; Fiber: 10g; Cholesterol: 0mg; Sodium: 710mg

Simple Salmon Burgers

SERVES 4 | **PREP TIME:** 10 minutes | **COOK TIME:** 10 minutes

For a nutritious and tasty twist, swap your usual ground beef for heart-healthy omega 3–rich salmon. These easy salmon burgers make for a light dinner you can have ready in under 30 minutes on busy weeknights. To save on carbs, skip the bun and serve the patties over a bed of salad greens lightly seasoned with vinegar and oil.

2 (6-ounce) cans boneless skinless salmon

1 large egg

½ cup whole-wheat bread crumbs

2 garlic cloves, minced

Juice of 1 lemon

1 tablespoon whole-grain or Dijon mustard

¼ teaspoon salt

¼ teaspoon freshly ground black pepper

1 tablespoon extra-virgin olive oil

4 whole-wheat hamburger buns

Lettuce, for serving

Sliced tomato, for serving

Mayonnaise, for serving

1. In a large bowl, stir together the salmon, egg, bread crumbs, garlic, lemon juice, mustard, salt, and pepper. Form the mixture into 4 patties.

2. In a large skillet over medium-high heat, heat the olive oil.

3. Add the patties and cook for 4 to 5 minutes per side, until golden brown.

4. Serve on the buns, topped with lettuce, tomato, and mayonnaise.

> **MAKE-AHEAD TIP:** Prepare the burgers the night before and refrigerate until ready to cook.

PER SERVING: Calories: 321; Total fat: 16g; Saturated fat: 3g; Protein: 22g; Carbs: 23g; Sugar: 4g; Fiber: 4g; Cholesterol: 95mg; Sodium: 419mg

Salmon and Veggie Bake

SERVES 4 | **PREP TIME:** 15 minutes | **COOK TIME:** 20 to 22 minutes

When you're short on time and dinner ideas, this protein-packed recipe is your ticket. You can save even more time by chopping the veggies the night before and preparing a healthy side such as Simple Brown Rice (page 119), herbed roasted potatoes, or sautéed Brussels sprouts. Cleanup is a snap if you line the pan with parchment paper.

1 medium zucchini, chopped into 1-inch pieces

1 red bell pepper, chopped into 1-inch pieces

1 medium onion, cut into wedges

2 tablespoons extra-virgin olive oil, divided

½ teaspoon salt, divided

½ teaspoon freshly ground black pepper, divided

3 garlic cloves, minced

2 teaspoons Dijon mustard

Juice of 1 lemon

1 pound salmon fillet, cut into 4 pieces

1. Preheat the oven to 425° F.

2. In a large bowl, combine the zucchini, red bell pepper, and onion. Add 1 tablespoon of olive oil, and toss to coat. Season with ¼ teaspoon each of salt and pepper. Spread the vegetables on a large baking sheet in a single layer, and bake for 10 minutes.

3. In the same bowl, whisk the remaining 1 tablespoon of olive oil with the garlic, mustard, lemon juice, and remaining ¼ teaspoon each of salt and pepper. Divide the mixture among the salmon fillets, and rub it into the flesh.

4. Once the vegetables have cooked for 10 minutes, nestle the salmon fillets on top of them. Bake for 10 to 12 minutes more, until the salmon flakes easily with a fork and the vegetables are tender. Serve the salmon with the vegetables.

TECHNIQUE TIP: Zucchini and bell peppers are great for this recipe because they are quick cooking but still take a little longer than the salmon to cook through. Be sure to get them into the oven and prepare the seasonings for the salmon while they are cooking to make the best use of time.

PER SERVING: Calories: 247; Total fat: 14g; Saturated fat: 2g; Protein: 24g; Carbs: 8g; Sugar: 4g; Fiber: 2g; Cholesterol: 50mg; Sodium: 379mg

Baked Parmesan-Crusted Halibut

SERVES 4 | **PREP TIME:** 10 minutes | **COOK TIME:** 15 minutes

For those who don't like the strong flavor of most oily ocean fish, halibut is for you. The mild, sweet taste of this white fish brings omega-3s to the table—and halibut is also an excellent source of protein, potassium, and niacin. The crunchy panko bread crumb coating is seasoned with Parmesan cheese and garlic powder and enhances the halibut's flavor. To achieve a crispy crust on both top and bottom, place the fish on a rack atop your baking sheet.

Nonstick cooking spray

½ cup whole-wheat panko bread crumbs

¼ cup shredded Parmesan cheese

1 tablespoon minced fresh parsley leaves

½ teaspoon garlic powder

½ teaspoon salt

¼ teaspoon freshly ground black pepper

Juice of ½ lemon

1 tablespoon extra-virgin olive oil

1 pound halibut fillet

1. Preheat the oven to 450° F. Place a rack on a baking sheet, and lightly spray with cooking spray.

2. On a large plate, combine the panko, Parmesan, parsley, garlic powder, salt, and pepper, and mix well.

3. Pour the lemon juice and olive oil over both sides of the halibut, and press the halibut into the coating mixture. Flip the fish, and press the coating onto the other side.

4. Transfer the fish to the prepared rack on the baking sheet, and lightly spray the top of the fish with cooking spray. Bake for 12 to 15 minutes, until the fish flakes easily with a fork, and serve.

INGREDIENT TIP: Panko bread crumbs are Japanese-style bread crumbs that are lighter and airier than the Italian variety. If you can't find whole-wheat panko near you, it is readily available online.

PER SERVING: Calories: 194; Total fat: 8g; Saturated fat: 2g; Protein: 26g; Carbs: 5g; Sugar: 0g; Fiber: 1g; Cholesterol: 41mg; Sodium: 432mg

Chicken Zoodle Soup

SERVES 4 | **PREP TIME:** 15 minutes | **COOK TIME:** 20 minutes

Ever had zoodles? This take on chicken noodle soup is a fun way to add extra veggies to your daily diet. If you already have a spiralizer, you're in business, but these zucchini noodles can also be made using a peeler, mandoline, or knife. This might become your go-to chicken soup.

1 tablespoon extra-virgin olive oil

2 celery stalks, chopped

2 carrots, chopped

1 onion, chopped

3 garlic cloves, chopped

8 ounces boneless skinless chicken breast, sliced thinly against the grain

4 cups low-sodium chicken broth

½ teaspoon chopped fresh thyme

½ teaspoon salt

¼ teaspoon freshly ground black pepper

2 medium zucchini, spiralized

1. In a large pot over medium-high heat, heat the olive oil.

2. Add the celery, carrots, and onion, and sauté for 5 to 7 minutes, until the onion softens.

3. Add the garlic, and cook for 30 seconds, until fragrant.

4. Add the chicken and cook, stirring, for 2 to 3 minutes, until just browned.

5. Stir in the chicken broth, thyme, salt, and pepper, and bring to a boil. Reduce the heat to maintain a simmer, and cook for 5 to 7 minutes, until the chicken is cooked through and the vegetables are tender.

6. Add the spiralized zucchini. Cook for 1 to 2 minutes more, until the zucchini is heated through, and serve.

MAKE-AHEAD TIP: Make the zucchini noodles the night before so prep time is reduced when you are ready to get cooking.

PER SERVING: Calories: 197; Total fat: 8g; Saturated fat: 2g; Protein: 20g; Carbs: 11g; Sugar: 5g; Fiber: 3g; Cholesterol: 50mg; Sodium: 449mg

Thai-Style Chicken Soup

SERVES 4 | **PREP TIME:** 10 minutes | **COOK TIME:** 15 minutes

This recipe features gluten-free rice noodles, curry paste, and coconut and will soon become a favorite. The coconut milk (you can use lite or full fat) adds a creamy, sweet, cooling counterpoint to the red curry paste. Use thin vermicelli rice noodles for this quick-cooking meal. And for an extra special garnish, top off your bowl with a couple of avocado slices for a dash of healthy monounsaturated fat.

1 tablespoon vegetable oil

1 small onion, thinly sliced

2 garlic cloves, minced

2 tablespoons red curry paste

4 cups low-sodium chicken broth

1 (15-ounce) can lite coconut milk

1½ cups sugar snap or snow peas, sliced lengthwise

4 ounces vermicelli rice noodles, broken into pieces

1 pound boneless skinless chicken breast, thinly sliced

1 tablespoon fish sauce

2 teaspoons brown sugar

Juice of 1 lime

1 lime, cut into wedges

Handful fresh basil leaves, chopped

1. In a large pot over medium-high heat, heat the vegetable oil.

2. Add the onion, and cook for 5 to 7 minutes, until softened and starting to brown.

3. Add the garlic and curry paste, and cook, stirring, for about 1 minute, until fragrant.

4. Stir in the chicken broth and coconut milk, and bring to a boil. Reduce the heat to maintain a simmer, and add the peas and noodles. Cook for about 3 minutes, until the noodles are just barely tender.

5. Add the chicken and simmer for 3 minutes, until cooked through.

6. Season with the fish sauce, brown sugar, and lime juice. Divide among bowls and serve with lime wedges and topped with basil.

INGREDIENT TIP: Red curry paste is typically available in the Asian section of most grocery stores. If you shop at an Asian grocery, you will notice there are many different types of curry paste—green, yellow, Panang, and Massaman—just to name a few. Once you taste this with the red curry, try another!

PER SERVING: Calories: 372; Total fat: 13g; Saturated fat: 6g; Protein: 33g; Carbs: 32g; Sugar: 3g; Fiber: 2g; Cholesterol: 65mg; Sodium: 912mg

Herb-Roasted Chicken Breast

SERVES 4 TO 6 | **PREP TIME:** 5 minutes | **COOK TIME:** 25 minutes

You know how bland, dry, overcooked chicken is no one's favorite? This recipe takes care of that. This easy meal uses key herbs and spices to create extremely juicy, flavorful chicken your family will love. Choose chicken breasts of equal size so they cook more evenly, and serve with a colorful side of steamed veggies such as asparagus, broccoli, or carrots.

1 tablespoon extra-virgin olive oil

1 teaspoon chopped fresh thyme

½ teaspoon dried oregano

½ teaspoon garlic powder

½ teaspoon onion powder

½ teaspoon salt

4 boneless skinless chicken breasts

1. Preheat the oven to 400° F.

2. In a small bowl, stir together the olive oil, thyme, oregano, garlic powder, onion powder, and salt.

3. Place the chicken breasts on a baking sheet or in a baking dish, and rub both sides with the herb mixture. Leave a couple of inches between each breast. Bake for 20 to 25 minutes, until the juices run clear and the internal temperature measures 165° F on an instant-read thermometer.

4. Let the chicken rest for 5 minutes before slicing and serving.

TECHNIQUE TIP: When cooking chicken breasts, which tend to dry out easily, having uniformly sized pieces helps with even cooking. If any of your chicken breasts are thicker than about ¾ inch, place them on a cutting board, cover with plastic wrap, and pound with a kitchen mallet until about ¾ inch thick.

PER SERVING: Calories: 153; Total fat: 5g; Saturated fat: 1g; Protein: 26g; Carbs: 1g; Sugar: 0g; Fiber: 0g; Cholesterol: 65mg; Sodium: 366mg

Turkey Meat Loaf

SERVES 6 | **PREP TIME:** 15 minutes, plus 10 minutes to stand | **COOK TIME:** 1 hour

Meat loaf may not be the sexiest of dishes, but when it comes to comfort food, it's the best. This recipe cuts way down on the fat by substituting ground turkey for ground beef. Prep and refrigerate this dish the night before, and you'll have dinner for the next evening meal ready to cook and eat. For an additional nutritional punch, experiment by adding grated zucchini or chopped shiitake mushrooms to the mix.

Nonstick cooking spray

1 tablespoon extra-virgin olive oil

1 onion, chopped

3 garlic cloves, minced

1½ pounds ground turkey

½ cup whole-wheat bread crumbs

1 large egg

1 teaspoon salt

½ teaspoon freshly ground black pepper

¼ cup ketchup

1. Preheat the oven to 350° F. Lightly coat an 8-by-4-inch loaf pan with cooking spray. Set aside.

2. In a small skillet over medium heat, heat the olive oil.

3. Add the onion and garlic, and sauté for 3 to 5 minutes, until the onion is softened. Remove from the heat, transfer to a large bowl, and let cool for about 5 minutes.

4. Once cooled, add the ground turkey, bread crumbs, egg, salt, and pepper. Mix well to combine. Press the mixture into the prepared loaf pan, and spread the ketchup over the top of the loaf. Bake for 50 to 55 minutes, until the internal temperature measures 165° F on an instant-read thermometer.

5. Remove from the oven and let stand for about 10 minutes before slicing into 6 pieces and serving.

INGREDIENT TIP: If you can't find whole-wheat bread crumbs at the grocery store, make your own! Save the ends of bread in the freezer in a bag, and when you need them, let thaw until you are able to break into pieces and process in a food processor into crumbs.

PER SERVING: Calories: 187; Total fat: 6g; Saturated fat: 1g; Protein: 28g; Carbs: 7g; Sugar: 3g; Fiber: 1g; Cholesterol: 93mg; Sodium: 620mg

Greek-Style Turkey Burgers

SERVES 4 | **PREP TIME:** 10 minutes | **COOK TIME:** 10 minutes

You may never go back to a regular hamburger again after having these Mediterranean burgers. Light and flavorful, the feta cheese does its job of keeping the meat moist. (Turkey tends to dry out more quickly than beef, so this is a tasty fix.) Top your turkey burger with the mint-yogurt sauce, lettuce, tomato, and cucumber, and you'll have a beautiful blend of mouthwatering flavors. To make it extra low-carb, forgo the buns.

¼ cup finely chopped red onion

¼ cup crumbled feta cheese

½ teaspoon dried oregano

1 pound ground turkey breast

1 teaspoon salt, divided

Freshly ground black pepper

1 tablespoon extra-virgin olive oil

½ cup plain nonfat Greek yogurt

1 tablespoon chopped fresh mint

1 garlic clove, minced

4 whole-wheat hamburger buns

Cucumber slices, for serving

Tomato slices, for serving

Lettuce leaves, for serving

1. In a small bowl, stir together the onion, feta, and oregano until well combined.

2. Form the ground turkey into 4 patties, and use a spoon to make an indent in the center of each. Place 2 tablespoons of the feta mixture in the indent in each patty. Fold the edges of the burgers over the filling, pressing to enclose, and flatten the burgers. Season the patties with ½ teaspoon of the salt and some pepper.

3. In a large skillet over medium heat, heat the olive oil.

4. Add the burgers, and cook for 5 minutes per side, flipping once, until browned and cooked through.

5. In a small bowl, whisk the yogurt, mint, garlic, and the remaining ½ teaspoon of salt.

6. Serve the burgers on the buns, topped with a dollop of the yogurt as well as the cucumber, tomato, and lettuce slices.

MAKE-AHEAD TIP: Make the patties the night before and reheat for lunch or dinner in the microwave for 1 to 2 minutes before topping with the yogurt sauce and vegetables.

PER SERVING: Calories: 295; Total fat: 8g; Saturated fat: 2g; Protein: 34g; Carbs: 23g; Sugar: 6g; Fiber: 4g; Cholesterol: 79mg; Sodium: 893mg

Asian-Style Chicken Wraps

SERVES 4 | **PREP TIME:** 10 minutes | **COOK TIME:** 10 minutes

You know those summer days when it's too hot to turn on the oven? This no-oven recipe is quick, easy, and best of all, tastes divine. Prep time can be even faster if you use preshredded carrots and cabbage (found in the produce section). Consider using a whole-wheat tortilla to make your meal a little more filling, or use a lettuce wrap. Either way, you'll have a delicious meal ready in no time flat.

¼ cup creamy peanut butter

2 tablespoons soy sauce

2 tablespoons honey

1 tablespoon minced peeled fresh ginger

1 tablespoon freshly squeezed lime juice

1 tablespoon extra-virgin olive oil

1 pound boneless skinless chicken breast, cut into bite-size pieces

1 cup shredded carrot

½ cup shredded cabbage

¼ cup sliced scallion, white and green parts

1 head red or green lettuce, leaves separated and washed

¼ cup salted peanuts

Handful chopped fresh cilantro

1. In a small bowl, whisk the peanut butter, soy sauce, honey, ginger, and lime juice. Set aside.

2. In a large skillet over medium-high heat, heat the olive oil.

3. Add the chicken, and cook for 3 to 5 minutes, until the pieces are cooked through. Transfer to a medium bowl, and toss with half of the peanut butter sauce.

4. Return the skillet to the heat, and add the carrot, cabbage, and scallion. Sauté for 1 to 2 minutes, until heated through and the cabbage wilts slightly. Remove from the skillet.

5. To serve, fill the lettuce leaves with a scoop of chicken and top with a scoop of the cabbage mixture. Garnish with peanuts and cilantro, and serve with the remaining sauce on the side.

PER SERVING: Calories: 361; Total fat: 18g; Saturated fat: 3g; Protein: 34g; Carbs: 21g; Sugar: 14g; Fiber: 3g; Cholesterol: 65mg; Sodium: 625mg

Chicken Shepherd's Pie

SERVES 6 | **PREP TIME:** 15 minutes, plus 10 minutes to rest | **COOK TIME:** 45 minutes

Warm your family with this easy remake of a favorite dish, featuring tender chicken, carrots, celery, and spinach. If you like, add ½ cup shredded cheese on top. Be sure to cook the cauliflower until really tender so it mashes and blends well with the potato. To complete this meal, consider a side salad with Balsamic Vinaigrette (page 113).

1 large baking potato, halved

3 cups chopped cauliflower

¼ cup unsweetened almond milk

1 tablespoon butter

½ teaspoon salt, divided

Freshly ground black pepper

1 tablespoon extra-virgin olive oil

2 celery stalks, chopped into ½-inch pieces

2 carrots, chopped into ½-inch pieces

1 onion, chopped

3 garlic cloves, minced

½ teaspoon dried thyme

2 tablespoons whole-wheat flour

1 cup low-sodium chicken or vegetable broth

2 cups chopped cooked chicken breast

2 cups packed sliced fresh spinach leaves

1. Bring a medium pot of water to boil over high heat. Add the potato, and cook for 5 minutes. Add the cauliflower, and continue to cook for 7 to 10 minutes more, until both are soft. Drain. When cool enough to handle, slide the skin off the potato and discard the skin. Using a potato masher or immersion blender, mash the potato and cauliflower together.

2. Add the almond milk, butter, ¼ teaspoon of the salt, and season with pepper. Stir to combine, and set aside.

3. Preheat the oven to 350°F.

4. In a large skillet over medium-high heat, heat the olive oil.

5. Add the celery, carrots, onion, garlic, and thyme, and sauté for 6 to 8 minutes, until the vegetables are just softened.

6. Stir in the flour, and cook for about 30 seconds.

7. Pour in the chicken broth, and stir to combine. Add the chicken, and bring the mixture to a simmer. Cook for 3 to 4 minutes, until the broth thickens.

8. Stir in the spinach, and transfer the mixture to a round or square 9-inch baking dish. Top with the mashed potato-cauliflower mixture, and bake for 15 minutes, until the top is lightly browned and the liquids are bubbling.

9. Let rest for 10 minutes before serving.

INGREDIENT TIP: If you don't have cooked chicken on hand, chop about 2 cups of chicken breast and cook it before the vegetables in ½ tablespoon of olive oil until cooked through. Set aside until ready to add in step 7.

PER SERVING: Calories: 211; Total fat: 6g; Saturated fat: 2g; Protein: 18g; Carbs: 21g; Sugar: 4g; Fiber: 4g; Cholesterol: 41mg; Sodium: 429mg

Chicken Breast and Veggie Bake

SERVES 4 | **PREP TIME:** 15 minutes | **COOK TIME:** 25 minutes

Healthy, easy, and delicious—the three basic qualities of a perfect weeknight meal! This dish redefines the meaning of "fast food." It's quick and simple, but loaded with health-promoting nutrients. You can customize the recipe to include your favorite veggies, too.

¼ cup red wine vinegar

2 tablespoons extra-virgin olive oil

1 teaspoon fresh thyme or ½ teaspoon dried thyme

½ teaspoon salt

Freshly ground black pepper

1 pound boneless skinless chicken breasts, halved lengthwise

1 head broccoli, separated into florets

1 red bell pepper, cut into strips

1 red onion, cut into wedges

8 ounces cremini mushrooms

1. Preheat the oven to 400° F. Line a baking sheet with parchment paper. Set aside.

2. In a small bowl, whisk the vinegar, olive oil, thyme, salt, and some pepper.

3. Place the chicken in a shallow dish, and pour half of the marinade over the chicken, flipping it to coat.

4. In a large bowl, toss the broccoli, red bell pepper, red onion, and mushrooms with the remaining marinade, being sure to coat all the vegetables. Transfer the vegetables to the prepared baking sheet.

5. Place the chicken breasts on top of the vegetables, and pour any remaining marinade over the chicken and vegetables. Bake for 20 to 25 minutes, depending on the thickness of the chicken breasts, until the chicken is cooked through and measures 165° F on an instant-read thermometer. Serve the chicken with the vegetables.

MAKE-AHEAD TIP: Marinate the meat for up to 8 hours in advance.

PER SERVING: Calories: 242; Total fat: 9g; Saturated fat: 1g; Protein: 30g; Carbs: 12g; Sugar: 5g; Fiber: 3g; Cholesterol: 65mg; Sodium: 394mg

Bean and Beef Taco Wraps

SERVES 4 | **PREP TIME:** 10 minutes | **COOK TIME:** 15 minutes

These appetizing wraps are sure to please everyone at the table. Use ground round beef, which has a lower fat content than ground chuck but still has all the flavor. The fiber in black beans adds bulk while also lowering fat. Whole-wheat tortillas are a traditional way of eating these wraps, but you can make them lighter by serving on lettuce leaves. Round out the meal with sliced apples and steamed carrots.

8 ounces lean ground beef

½ cup cooked black beans

½ cup salsa, divided

1 teaspoon onion powder

1 teaspoon chili powder

¼ teaspoon garlic powder

Freshly ground black pepper

4 whole-wheat flour tortillas

1 cup finely sliced lettuce, divided

¼ cup shredded Cheddar cheese, divided

1. In a large skillet over medium-high heat, cook the beef for about 7 minutes, until browned and cooked through. Drain.

2. Add the black beans, ¼ cup of salsa, and the onion powder, chili powder, and garlic powder. Season with pepper, and stir to combine. Bring the mixture to a boil, reduce the heat to low, and simmer for 5 minutes.

3. Into each tortilla, spoon one-quarter of the meat mixture, ¼ cup of lettuce, 1 tablespoon of cheese, and 1 tablespoon of the remaining salsa, and serve.

MAKE-AHEAD TIP: The meat mixture can be made up to 3 days in advance. When ready to serve, simply reheat and fill the tortillas, top with lettuce and cheese, and enjoy.

PER SERVING: Calories: 318; Total fat: 9g; Saturated fat: 4g; Protein: 24g; Carbs: 34g; Sugar: 2g; Fiber: 8g; Cholesterol: 55mg; Sodium: 455mg

Slow Cooker Pulled Pork Sandwiches

SERVES 8 | **PREP TIME:** 5 minutes | **COOK TIME:** 6 to 8 hours on low or 4 to 5 hours on high

What would we do without our slow cookers? Cooks all day while the cook's away—or so the saying goes. There's no easier way to prepare dinner than throwing it all into the slow cooker in the morning so it's ready when you walk in the door that night. This super simple pulled pork recipe is done when you can shred it easily with two forks. Served on rolls or by itself, this tantalizing recipe goes great with a side of Quick Coleslaw (page 103) or a three-bean salad.

Nonstick cooking spray

2 cups barbecue sauce (look for a low-sugar variety)

1 medium onion, chopped

2 garlic cloves, minced

2 tablespoons honey

1 teaspoon salt

½ teaspoon freshly ground black pepper

2 pounds boneless pork loin, cut into 3 or 4 pieces

8 whole-wheat rolls

1. Spray the slow cooker insert lightly with cooking spray.

2. In the cooker, stir together the barbecue sauce, onion, garlic, honey, salt, and pepper.

3. Add the pork pieces, and turn to coat with the sauce.

4. Cover the cooker, and cook for 6 to 8 hours on low, or 4 to 5 hours on high, until the pork is very tender.

5. Using two forks, shred the pork and mix well with the sauce in the cooker. Serve on the rolls.

PER SERVING: Calories: 297; Total fat: 9g; Saturated fat: 3g; Protein: 27g; Carbs: 28g; Sugar: 8g; Fiber: 3g; Cholesterol: 60mg; Sodium: 550mg

Mushroom and Beef Burgers

SERVES 4 | **PREP TIME:** 10 minutes | **COOK TIME:** 20 minutes

A really good burger is something we all crave now and then. To keep fat and calories under control, use ground round beef and form a 4-ounce patty (about the size and thickness of the palm of your hand). The mushrooms keep it lean without losing any of the meaty flavor you expect. Grilling or broiling is also an acceptable lean-cooking method for these.

8 ounces cremini mushrooms

1 tablespoon extra-virgin olive oil

1 onion, finely chopped

3 garlic cloves, minced

8 ounces lean ground beef

½ teaspoon salt

¼ teaspoon freshly ground black pepper

4 whole-wheat hamburger buns

Ketchup, for serving

Mustard, for serving

Lettuce leaves, for serving

1. In a food processor, pulse the mushrooms a few times until coarsely ground.

2. In a large skillet over medium-high heat, heat the olive oil.

3. Add the ground mushrooms, onion, and garlic, and sauté for 8 to 10 minutes, until the vegetables soften and the liquid evaporates. Remove from the pan, and cool completely.

4. In a large bowl, combine the ground beef, cooled mushroom mixture, salt, and pepper. Mix well. Form the meat mixture into 4 patties.

5. Return the skillet to medium-high heat. Add the patties, and cook for 3 to 5 minutes per side, until cooked to your desired level of doneness.

6. Serve on the buns, topped with ketchup, mustard, and lettuce leaves.

PER SERVING: Calories: 311; Total fat: 13g; Saturated fat: 3g; Protein: 21g; Carbs: 29g; Sugar: 9g; Fiber: 4g; Cholesterol: 48mg; Sodium: 629mg

Herb-Crusted Pork Tenderloin

SERVES 4 | **PREP TIME:** 10 minutes | **COOK TIME:** 25 minutes

This lean cut of pork is widely available and very easy and quick to cook. The moist meat gets a flavor boost from the herbs and spices, while the whole-wheat panko bread crumb coating adds crunchiness. Serve it with Simple Brown Rice (page 119) and roasted veggies, such as asparagus and red bell peppers.

1 teaspoon ground mustard

1 teaspoon salt

½ teaspoon freshly ground black pepper

1 (1-pound) pork tenderloin, trimmed

2 tablespoons extra-virgin olive oil, divided

1 cup whole-wheat panko bread crumbs

2 teaspoons minced fresh thyme

1 garlic clove, minced

½ teaspoon ground cumin

1 tablespoon Dijon mustard

1. Preheat the oven to 425° F.

2. In a small bowl, stir together the dry mustard, salt, and pepper, and rub the spices over the tenderloin.

3. In a large cast iron skillet or other oven-safe skillet over medium-high heat, heat 1 tablespoon of olive oil.

4. Add the pork and sear on all sides, about 2 minutes per side, until browned.

5. Meanwhile, in a small bowl, stir together the bread crumbs, thyme, garlic, cumin, and remaining 1 tablespoon of olive oil.

6. Spread the mustard on the top of the tenderloin, and press the bread crumb mixture into it. Transfer the skillet to the oven and bake for 12 to 15 minutes, until the internal temperature measures 140° F on an instant-read thermometer and the juices run clear.

7. Let rest for 5 minutes before slicing and serving.

PER SERVING: Calories: 301; Total fat: 13g; Saturated fat: 2g; Protein: 26g; Carbs: 21g; Sugar: 1g; Fiber: 2g; Cholesterol: 0mg; Sodium: 220mg

Flank Steak with Chimichurri

SERVES 4 | **PREP TIME:** 15 minutes | **COOK TIME:** 10 minutes

If flank steak is served, especially with this super tasty and incredibly easy chimichurri, expect a rush to the dinner table. A lean, nutritious, boneless cut with lots of intense beef flavor, flank steak has more protein per ounce (about 8 grams) than other steak cuts like porterhouse or rib eye. Remember to cut across the grain when serving, which yields a more tender piece of meat.

FOR THE CHIMICHURRI

¼ cup packed fresh parsley leaves

¼ cup packed fresh cilantro leaves

¼ cup chopped red onion

1 garlic clove, peeled

2 tablespoons extra-virgin olive oil

2 tablespoons water

1 tablespoon apple cider vinegar

¼ teaspoon salt

Freshly ground black pepper

Red pepper flakes

FOR THE FLANK STEAK

1 pound flank steak, trimmed

1 teaspoon salt

½ teaspoon garlic powder

Freshly ground black pepper

TO MAKE THE CHIMICHURRI

In a food processor, combine the parsley, cilantro, red onion, garlic, olive oil, water, vinegar, and salt. Pulse a few times until just combined. Season with black pepper and red pepper flakes, and set aside.

TO MAKE THE FLANK STEAK

1. Season both sides of the steak with the salt, garlic powder, and some black pepper.

2. Heat a large cast iron skillet over high heat.

3. Add the steak to the hot pan, and cook for 3 to 5 minutes per side, flipping once, until medium-rare. Transfer to a cutting board and let rest for 5 minutes. Cut into thin strips across the grain, and serve topped with the chimichurri sauce.

VARIATION TIP: Flank steak is also great on the grill. Cook the steak directly over medium-hot coals for 3 to 5 minutes per side to add a smoky flavor.

PER SERVING: Calories: 263; Total fat: 17g; Saturated fat: 1g; Protein: 25g; Carbs: 1g; Sugar: 1g; Fiber: 0g; Cholesterol: 0mg; Sodium: 732mg

Rosemary-Crusted Lamb

SERVES 4 | **PREP TIME:** 5 minutes, plus 30 minutes to marinate | **COOK TIME:** 20 minutes

I don't believe there is a simpler, or more show-stopping, lamb recipe than this one. It may not be as popular as beef, chicken, or fish, but lamb is an incredibly nutritious meat that's not to be overlooked. Rich in protein, it is also a good source of vitamin B_{12} and iron, important for the production of red blood cells. While lamb is often associated with Easter and Passover celebrations, it's perfect any time of the year for a special dinner. To complete the meal, consider serving Cauli-Couscous (page 108) and braised green beans.

3 garlic cloves, minced

2 tablespoons extra-virgin olive oil

2 teaspoons chopped fresh rosemary

1 teaspoon salt

½ teaspoon freshly ground black pepper

8 (3- to 4-ounce) lamb rib chops, trimmed

1. In a small bowl, stir together the garlic, olive oil, rosemary, salt, and pepper. Spread the mixture onto the lamb chops, and let rest for 30 minutes.

2. Heat a large cast iron skillet over medium-high heat. Press the rosemary and garlic onto the chops, and, working in batches, gently place the chops in the hot pan. Cook for 4 to 5 minutes per side, flipping once, until medium-rare. Keep warm while cooking the remaining chops, and serve.

PER SERVING: Calories: 396; Total fat: 29g; Saturated fat: 13g; Protein: 30g; Carbs: 1g; Sugar: 0g; Fiber: 0g; Cholesterol: 98mg; Sodium: 668mg

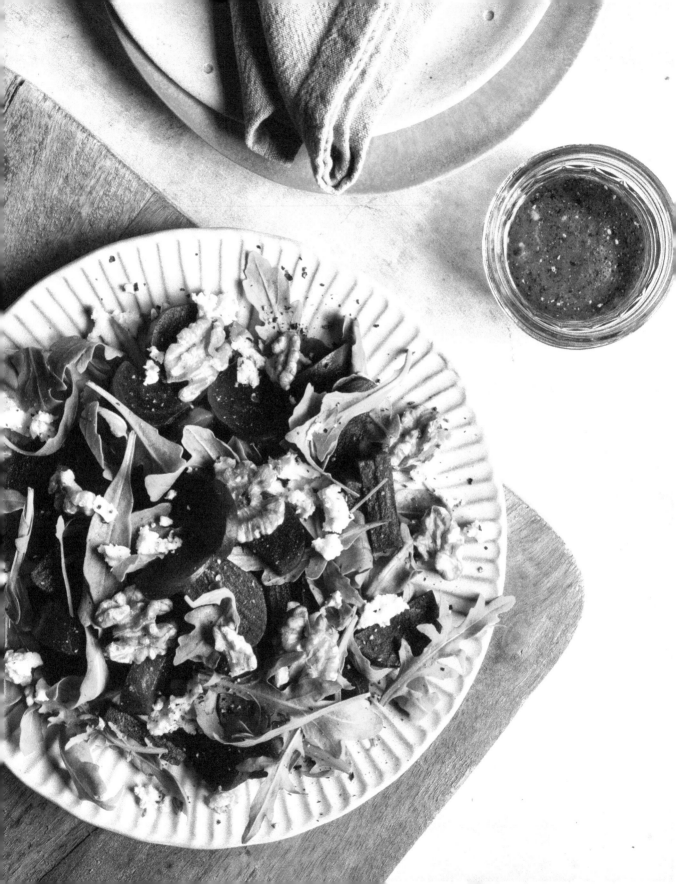

— SIX —

Sides & Staples

◀ ROASTED BEET SALAD, PAGE 107

Vegetable Rolls with Dipping Sauce

SERVES 4 | **PREP TIME:** 15 minutes

We're always told to eat more veggies, and here's a good way to do it. Great as a snack, these low-carb vegetable rolls are loaded with antioxidant-rich nutrients that provide a quick pick-me-up when hunger strikes. Collard leaves provide the perfect wrap around whatever veggies you choose—feel free to swap out those listed for your favorites.

FOR THE VEGETABLE ROLLS

1 cup shredded
Napa cabbage

1 cup shredded carrot

1 cup bean sprouts

1 red bell pepper, sliced

4 scallions, green and
white parts, sliced

¼ cup chopped
fresh cilantro

Salt

Freshly ground
black pepper

8 large collard green leaves

FOR THE DIPPING SAUCE

½ cup peanut butter

2 tablespoons soy sauce

1 tablespoon rice vinegar

1 teaspoon honey

3 garlic cloves, minced

TO MAKE THE VEGETABLE ROLLS

1. In a large bowl, toss together the cabbage, carrot, bean sprouts, red bell pepper, scallions, and cilantro. Season lightly with salt and pepper.

2. Fold 1 collard leaf in half along the stem, stem facing out. Holding the leaf with one hand, pull the stem up and away using your opposite hand. Repeat with the remaining collard greens.

3. On top of each collard leaf, place about ½ cup of the vegetable mixture, fold the sides in, and roll the leaf up like a burrito. Place on a serving platter, seam-side down. Repeat with the remaining leaves and vegetable mixture.

TO MAKE THE DIPPING SAUCE

In a small bowl, whisk the peanut butter, soy sauce, vinegar, honey, and garlic. Serve with the vegetable rolls for dipping.

PER SERVING: Calories: 271; Total fat: 17g; Saturated fat: 4g; Protein: 13g; Carbs: 23g; Sugar: 10g; Fiber: 5g; Cholesterol: 0mg; Sodium: 705mg

Kale Salad with Avocado Dressing

SERVES 6 | **PREP TIME:** 10 minutes

Maybe you like kale and maybe you don't. But this dark leafy green salad—I recommend mild-tasting baby kale—will be a year-round lunch favorite. Between fiber- and potassium-rich kale (great for blood pressure) and heart-healthy fats found in avocados and cashews, this salad does its part in keeping you full and satisfied for hours. To prevent browning of the avocado, don't peel until ready to use.

6 cups chopped kale

1 cup finely chopped red bell pepper

1 bunch scallions, white and green parts, finely chopped

1 avocado, pitted and peeled

½ cup raw cashews

3 garlic cloves, peeled

Juice of ½ lemon

¼ cup extra-virgin olive oil

Salt

Freshly ground black pepper

1. In a large bowl, toss together the kale, red bell pepper, and scallions.

2. In a high-speed blender or food processor, combine the avocado, cashews, garlic, lemon juice, and olive oil, and process until smooth. Add up to ½ cup of water as needed to create a pourable dressing. Season with salt and pepper. Pour the dressing over the kale, mix well, and serve.

PER SERVING: Calories: 232; Total fat: 18g; Saturated fat: 3g; Protein: 5g; Carbs: 16g; Sugar: 2g; Fiber: 4g; Cholesterol: 0mg; Sodium: 64mg

Cucumber Salad

SERVES 4 | **PREP TIME:** 10 minutes

There are few side dishes as good as a Cucumber Salad. Fresh, filling, and flavorful, this salad is a snap to create. If you find your cucumbers on the seedy side, simply remove the excess seeds first. The secret to this salad's success is the sharp, tangy flavor of red wine vinegar—one of the most popular vinegars found in kitchen pantries.

2 medium cucumbers, peeled and chopped

1 cup cherry tomatoes, halved

½ red onion, thinly sliced

2 tablespoons red wine vinegar

2 tablespoons extra-virgin olive oil

¼ teaspoon dried oregano

¼ teaspoon salt, plus more as needed

Freshly ground black pepper

1. In a medium bowl, combine the cucumbers, tomatoes, and red onion.

2. In a small bowl, whisk the vinegar, olive oil, oregano, salt, and some pepper. Pour the vinaigrette over the vegetables, and toss to coat. Taste and season with more salt and pepper, if desired. Serve immediately, or refrigerate in an airtight container for 2 to 3 days.

PER SERVING: Calories: 98; Total fat: 7g; Saturated fat: 1g; Protein: 2g; Carbs: 9g; Sugar: 4g; Fiber: 2g; Cholesterol: 0mg; Sodium: 153mg

Quick Coleslaw

SERVES 4 | **PREP TIME:** 15 minutes

Coleslaw is one of the most underrated and overlooked healthy sides around. Packed with all sorts of health-boosting nutrients, from vitamins C and K to folate and fiber, this dairy-free coleslaw is much healthier than the typical varieties made with mayo. The combination of green and red cabbage along with carrots makes a nice pop of color for your plate.

¼ cup extra-virgin olive oil

Juice of 1 lemon

1 garlic clove, minced

½ teaspoon salt

2 cups finely sliced green cabbage

2 cups finely sliced red cabbage

1 cup shredded carrot

4 scallions, white and green parts, chopped

1. In a small bowl, whisk the olive oil, lemon juice, garlic, and salt. Set aside.

2. In a medium bowl, toss together the green and red cabbage, carrot, and scallions. Pour the dressing over the cabbage, and mix well to coat. Serve immediately or refrigerate for several hours before serving.

INGREDIENT TIP: If you don't think you'll eat the leftover cabbage, look in the refrigerated produce section for halved cabbages to minimize food waste.

PER SERVING: Calories: 146; Total fat: 13g; Saturated fat: 2g; Protein: 2g; Carbs: 8g; Sugar: 4g; Fiber: 3g; Cholesterol: 0mg; Sodium: 327mg

Creamy Tomato Soup

SERVES 4 | **PREP TIME:** 10 minutes | **COOK TIME:** 20 minutes

One of my personal year-round favorites is homemade tomato soup. Simmering oil, onions, garlic, and tomatoes fill my home with wonderful aromas as I eagerly anticipate a steaming hot bowl to eat. Made with readily available ingredients, it's easy to make and so smooth you'll never eat canned, sodium-laden tomato soup again. If you're feeding a larger crowd, it's easily doubled and makes great leftovers. Thinly sliced bread and a bowl of your favorite fruit complete this healthy meal.

1 tablespoon extra-virgin olive oil

½ onion, chopped

½ red bell pepper, chopped

3 garlic cloves, minced

1 (28-ounce) can no-salt-added whole tomatoes

1½ cups low-sodium vegetable broth

½ cup skim milk

½ teaspoon salt

¼ teaspoon freshly ground black pepper

2 tablespoons chopped fresh basil

¼ cup shredded Parmesan cheese (optional)

1. In a large pot over medium heat, heat the olive oil.

2. Increase the heat to medium-high, and add the onion and red bell pepper. Sauté for 3 to 5 minutes, until softened.

3. Add the garlic, and cook for 30 seconds more, until fragrant.

4. Stir in the tomatoes and their juices and the vegetable broth. Bring to a boil, reduce the heat to maintain a simmer, and cook for 10 minutes.

5. Using an immersion blender, purée the soup in the pot. Alternately, transfer the soup, in batches, to a regular blender, purée the soup, and return it to the pot.

6. Stir in the milk, salt, and pepper. Heat for about 1 minute, until heated through.

7. Stir in the basil and serve, topping each serving with 1 tablespoon of Parmesan (if using).

INGREDIENT TIP: Canned goods are loaded with sodium, including vegetables such as tomatoes and beans. When available, always select low-sodium or no-salt-added products and season foods yourself to better control your sodium intake.

PER SERVING (1½ CUPS): Calories: 103; Total fat: 4g; Saturated fat: 1g; Protein: 4g; Carbs: 14g; Sugar: 8g; Fiber: 4g; Cholesterol: 1mg; Sodium: 385mg

Creamy Broccoli Soup

SERVES 4 | **PREP TIME:** 5 minutes | **COOK TIME:** 15 minutes

Cream of broccoli soup is a staple. But if you find restaurant versions loaded with fat, here's a slimmed-down solution that's also extremely quick and easy to prepare. Within about 20 minutes, you'll have created a delightful calcium-rich, ultra-creamy soup. Perfect for a light lunch, this soup makes a great go-to when rushed for time.

3 small broccoli crowns, chopped

2 cups low-sodium vegetable broth

4 tablespoons butter

6 tablespoons whole-wheat flour

3 cups skim milk

½ teaspoon salt

¼ teaspoon freshly ground black pepper

1. In a large pot over high heat, combine the broccoli and vegetable broth, and bring to a boil. Reduce the heat to medium, cover the pot, and cook for 7 to 10 minutes, until tender.

2. Meanwhile, in a small saucepan over medium heat, melt the butter. Whisk in the flour and cook for about 1 minute, stirring constantly. While whisking continuously, slowly add the milk until it is all incorporated. Simmer briefly until just thickened.

3. Using an immersion blender, purée the soup in the pot. Alternately, transfer the soup, in batches, to a regular blender, purée the soup, and return it to the pot.

4. Stir the cream sauce into the soup, season with the salt and pepper, and serve.

VARIATION TIP: If you prefer broccoli-Cheddar soup, stir in about ½ cup shredded Cheddar cheese with the cream sauce to create an even more indulgent soup.

PER SERVING (1½ CUPS): Calories: 258; Total fat: 12g; Saturated fat: 7g; Protein: 12g; Carbs: 26g; Sugar: 11g; Fiber: 5g; Cholesterol: 34mg; Sodium: 550mg

Sautéed Greens

SERVES 4 | **PREP TIME:** 10 minutes | **COOK TIME:** 5 minutes

Too many of us are unsure of how to cook greens; by following these simple, step-by-step instructions, you'll be a kitchen pro quickly preparing nutrient-dense greens in no time. Whichever greens you like best, just remove the stem by folding the leaves in half, holding the leaves down with one hand, and pulling the stem away with the other. These delicious greens pair well with both vegetarian and meat-based meals.

2 tablespoons extra-virgin olive oil

3 garlic cloves, minced

1 pound kale, collard greens, or Swiss chard, stemmed and cut into ½-inch strips

Red wine vinegar, for seasoning

Salt

1. In a large skillet over medium-high heat, heat the olive oil.

2. Add the garlic and cook for 30 seconds, until fragrant.

3. Add the kale to the skillet, and stir well. Reduce the heat to medium-low and cover. Cook for 3 to 5 minutes, stirring occasionally, until the greens are tender.

4. Remove the lid, season with vinegar and salt, and serve.

PER SERVING: Calories: 86; Total fat: 7g; Saturated fat: 1g; Protein: 2g; Carbs: 5g; Sugar: 1g; Fiber: 2g; Cholesterol: 0mg; Sodium: 282mg

Roasted Beet Salad

SERVES 4 | **PREP TIME:** 10 minutes | **COOK TIME:** 1 hour 10 minutes

Freshly roasted beets are sure to delight. They're earthy and sweet and, when tossed with greens, feta cheese, walnuts, and vinaigrette, they make a perfect starter for a special meal. Roasting does take some time; to speed things up, roast the beets up to 2 days in advance and refrigerate until ready to use. Key to creating a masterpiece recipe is using good-quality balsamic vinegar—avoid any with lots of sugar.

6 medium beets, scrubbed, tops removed

¼ cup balsamic vinegar

¼ cup extra-virgin olive oil

1 teaspoon Dijon mustard

Salt

Freshly ground black pepper

¼ cup walnuts

6 ounces baby arugula

2 ounces feta cheese, crumbled

1. Preheat the oven to 400° F.

2. Wrap each beet tightly in aluminum foil, and arrange on a baking sheet. Roast for 45 to 60 minutes, depending on their size, until tender when pierced with a knife. Remove from the oven, carefully unwrap each beet, and let cool for 10 minutes.

3. Reduce the oven temperature to 350° F.

4. Meanwhile, in a medium bowl, whisk the vinegar, olive oil, and mustard. Season with salt and pepper.

5. On the same baking sheet, spread the walnuts in a single layer. Toast for 5 to 7 minutes, until lightly browned.

6. Using a small knife, peel and slice the beets, and place them in another medium bowl. Add half the vinaigrette, and toss to coat.

7. Add the arugula to the remaining vinaigrette, and toss to coat.

8. On a serving platter, arrange the arugula and top with the beets. Sprinkle the toasted walnuts and feta cheese over the top and serve.

TECHNIQUE TIP: Do not skip the baking sheet underneath the beets. Once tender, beets can get really juicy and drip in the oven, creating quite a mess if you don't have the baking sheet to catch the juices.

PER SERVING: Calories: 267; Total fat: 20g; Saturated fat: 4g; Protein: 7g; Carbs: 18g; Sugar: 14g; Fiber: 4g; Cholesterol: 13mg; Sodium: 339mg

Cauli-Couscous

SERVES 6 | **PREP TIME:** 10 minutes | **COOK TIME:** 5 minutes

It seems the chameleonlike qualities of cauliflower are never-ending. This recipe uses cauliflower to create a couscous-like side dish. Prep the cauliflower up to 2 days in advance, if you like, and be sure to put a lid on the skillet when steaming for just the right texture. Turmeric's anti-inflammatory and antioxidant powers meet with golden raisins for an outstanding combination of savory and sweet.

1 head cauliflower, cored and cut into florets

½ teaspoon salt

½ teaspoon ground turmeric

½ cup golden raisins

1. In a food processor, pulse the cauliflower several times until it resembles a coarse, couscous-like grain.

2. In a large skillet over medium-high heat, combine the cauliflower, salt, and turmeric. Add just enough water to cover the bottom of the pan. Bring to a simmer, reduce the heat to low, and cover the skillet. Steam for 5 minutes.

3. Remove the lid, and cook off any water remaining in the pan. Stir in the raisins and serve.

PER SERVING: Calories: 72; Total fat: 0g; Saturated fat: 0g; Protein: 3g; Carbs: 17g; Sugar: 11g; Fiber: 4g; Cholesterol: 0mg; Sodium: 237mg

Quinoa Pilaf

SERVES 6 | **PREP TIME:** 10 minutes, plus 10 minutes to rest | **COOK TIME:** 35 minutes

A great side dish can bring out the best in a meal. The quinoa craze is still going strong, and for good reason. Quinoa is a gluten-free, whole-grain seed resembling a grain that has enchanted the taste buds of many a cook. This recipe takes just a tad longer to cook, but once in the pot, it gives you 15 minutes of hands-off time. Toasting the almonds is a must for adding great flavor. If you're out of wine, use an extra ¼ cup of broth instead.

½ cup slivered almonds

1 tablespoon extra-virgin olive oil

½ onion, chopped

½ red bell pepper, chopped

1 cup quinoa, rinsed

¼ cup dry white wine

1¼ cups low-sodium vegetable broth

1 cucumber, peeled and finely chopped

Zest of 1 lemon

½ teaspoon salt

¼ teaspoon freshly ground black pepper

1. Preheat the oven to 350° F.

2. On a baking sheet, spread the almonds in a single layer. Toast for 5 to 7 minutes, until lightly toasted. Set aside.

3. Meanwhile, in a large pan or skillet over medium-high heat, heat the olive oil.

4. Add the onion, and sauté for about 2 minutes, until just starting to soften.

5. Add the red bell pepper, and cook for 5 minutes more, until the vegetables are tender.

6. Add the quinoa to the skillet, and cook for about 2 minutes, stirring constantly, until lightly toasted.

7. Stir in the wine and cook, stirring constantly, until evaporated, about 5 minutes.

8. Add the vegetable broth, and bring to a boil. Reduce the heat to maintain a simmer, cover the pan, and cook for 12 to 15 minutes, until all the liquid is evaporated. Turn off the heat and let sit for 10 minutes.

9. Add the cucumber, lemon zest, salt, and pepper, toss well to combine, and serve.

PER SERVING: Calories: 196; Total fat: 8g; Saturated fat: 1g; Protein: 7g; Carbs: 24g; Sugar: 2g; Fiber: 4g; Cholesterol: 0mg; Sodium: 212mg

Black Bean and Corn Salad

SERVES 5 | **PREP TIME:** 15 minutes

This salad is a crowd-pleaser, guaranteed. When you serve a hearty side that blends perfectly with meats and Mexican dishes alike, be prepared when everyone wants the recipe. Full of tantalizing flavors, it's great not only as a side but even for dipping chips and pita bread. The best thing about this recipe is there is no cooking involved—use canned black beans, and throw everything else together. Voilà—it's ready!

2 (15-ounce) cans reduced-sodium black beans, rinsed and drained

1 red bell pepper, chopped

1 cucumber, chopped

1 avocado, peeled, seeded, and chopped

1 cup fresh, frozen and thawed, or canned and drained corn

½ cup minced red onion

1 jalapeño pepper, seeded and minced

¼ cup chopped fresh cilantro

¼ cup extra-virgin olive oil

3 tablespoons freshly squeezed lime juice

1 teaspoon honey

1 teaspoon ground cumin

Salt

Freshly ground black pepper

1. In a large bowl, stir together the black beans, red bell pepper, cucumber, avocado, corn, red onion, jalapeño, and cilantro.

2. In a small bowl, whisk the olive oil, lime juice, honey, and cumin. Season with salt and pepper. Pour the dressing over the salad, mix well to coat, and serve.

INGREDIENT TIP: When using canned beans, always drain and rinse to remove additional sodium contained in the packing liquid.

PER SERVING: Calories: 313; Total fat: 19g; Saturated fat: 3g; Protein: 9g; Carbs: 32g; Sugar: 7g; Fiber: 11g; Cholesterol: 0mg; Sodium: 260mg

Sweet Potato Fries

SERVES 4 | **PREP TIME:** 10 minutes | **COOK TIME:** 25 minutes

If only all recipes were this easy and tasted this good. Naturally sweet and a great source of vitamins A and C, Sweet Potato Fries are a nice alternative to traditional fries. Dress them up a bit by adding the chopped leaves from a thyme or rosemary sprig before cooking. While these fries bake to perfection, grill some burgers or whip up another fantastic side dish.

1 pound sweet potatoes, cut lengthwise and then into strips

2 tablespoons extra-virgin olive oil

½ teaspoon salt

1. Preheat the oven to 425° F.

2. In a large bowl, combine the sweet potatoes, olive oil, and salt, and toss to coat.

3. Arrange the sweet potatoes on a baking sheet in a single layer. Bake for about 25 minutes, flipping once or twice during cooking, until the sweet potatoes are tender and crisp, and serve.

PREP TIP: Cutting uniformly sized fries means they cook and crisp evenly, so take the extra time to cut the sweet potatoes as uniformly as you can. Aim for ½-inch-thick fries. Sweet potatoes cook a bit quicker than white potatoes, and this size lets them cook through and crisp a bit in about 25 minutes.

PER SERVING: Calories: 158; Total fat: 7g; Saturated fat: 1g; Protein: 2g; Carbs: 23g; Sugar: 5g; Fiber: 3g; Cholesterol: 0mg; Sodium: 353mg

Polenta

SERVES 4 | **PREP TIME:** 5 minutes | **COOK TIME:** 20 minutes

Polenta may sound glamorous, but it's a wonderful gluten-free side dish requiring few ingredients. The secret to polenta that's thick and slightly sweet is cornmeal, broth, and butter. For an additional flavor boost, Parmesan cheese provides a delightfully savory note, making it taste like a much fancier dish. Not sure what to serve it with? Polenta pairs well with rich, savory dishes and is a good alternative to pasta. Try it with Sautéed Greens (page 106) or mushrooms, or even the omega-3–rich Salmon and Veggie Bake (page 82). Keep portion sizes in check, as corn is higher in carbs than some other sides.

2 cups low-sodium vegetable broth

2 cups water

1 teaspoon salt

1 cup yellow cornmeal

1 tablespoon butter

¼ cup shredded Parmesan cheese

1. In a medium saucepan over high heat, bring the vegetable broth and water to a boil. Add the salt, and slowly whisk in the cornmeal. Reduce the heat to low and cook for about 15 minutes, stirring regularly, until the polenta thickens and becomes tender.

2. Stir in the butter and Parmesan cheese until melted and serve.

PER SERVING: Calories: 166; Total fat: 6g; Saturated fat: 3g; Protein: 6g; Carbs: 24g; Sugar: 0g; Fiber: 2g; Cholesterol: 13mg; Sodium: 713mg

Balsamic Vinaigrette

MAKES ABOUT 1 CUP | **PREP TIME:** 5 minutes

Ditch the store-bought dressings for this easy Balsamic Vinaigrette, which may be the best you've ever had. The nice thing about vinaigrettes is how versatile they are. Swap out balsamic for red wine vinegar or even freshly squeezed lemon juice. No matter how you like it, this vinaigrette will become a staple in your fridge.

¾ cup extra-virgin olive oil

¼ cup balsamic vinegar

2 garlic cloves, minced

1 teaspoon Dijon mustard

½ teaspoon freshly ground black pepper

¼ teaspoon salt

In a small bowl or lidded jar, combine the olive oil, vinegar, garlic, mustard, pepper, and salt. Whisk to combine, or cover and shake until blended. Keep covered, and refrigerate for up to 1 month.

PER SERVING (2 TABLESPOONS): Calories: 171; Total fat: 19g; Saturated fat: 3g; Protein: 0g; Carbs: 2g; Sugar: 1g; Fiber: 0g; Cholesterol: 0mg; Sodium: 83mg

Creamy Ranch Dressing

SERVES 4 | **PREP TIME:** 10 minutes

I'll admit it: I like a good ranch dressing—who doesn't? But store-bought versions can be overly creamy and full of fat. To keep the creamy richness without the excess calories, make your own—with less fat yet tons of flavor thanks to the variety of herbs. For those of you who prefer a thicker dressing, add half the milk first and then adjust as desired.

¾ cup fat-free sour cream

½ cup plain nonfat Greek yogurt

Juice of ½ lemon

2 teaspoons dried chives

2 teaspoons dried parsley

1 teaspoon salt

1 teaspoon garlic powder

1 teaspoon onion powder

1 cup skim milk

Freshly ground black pepper

1. In a small bowl, stir together the sour cream and yogurt.

2. Add the lemon juice, chives, parsley, salt, garlic powder, and onion powder, and stir well to combine.

3. Whisk in the milk until smooth, and season with pepper. Transfer to a jar, cover, and refrigerate for up to 2 weeks.

PER SERVING: Calories: 91; Total fat: 0g; Saturated fat: 0g; Protein: 5g; Carbs: 14g; Sugar: 9g; Fiber: 1g; Cholesterol: 0mg; Sodium: 677mg

Mushroom Gravy

SERVES 6 | **PREP TIME:** 10 minutes | **COOK TIME:** 20 minutes

This Mushroom Gravy is meaty, rich tasting, and everything you want and expect from gravy. One unusual twist is the whole-wheat flour. Cook the flour when dry to add a bit of color as well as flavor to the gravy. A rule of thumb when making any gravy is, always use a whisk—otherwise you'll be making lumpy gravy!

2 tablespoons extra-virgin olive oil

1 onion, chopped

8 ounces sliced mushrooms

1 garlic clove, minced

¼ cup whole-wheat flour

2 cups low-sodium vegetable or chicken broth

½ teaspoon salt

½ teaspoon chopped fresh thyme, or ¼ teaspoon dried thyme

¼ teaspoon freshly ground black pepper

¼ cup skim milk

1. In a large skillet over medium-high heat, heat the olive oil.

2. Add the onion, and sauté for 3 to 5 minutes, until beginning to soften.

3. Add the mushrooms, and cook for 5 to 7 minutes, until browned and the liquid has evaporated.

4. Add the garlic, and sauté for 30 seconds, until fragrant.

5. Add the flour and cook, stirring constantly, for 1 to 2 minutes.

6. While whisking, slowly pour in the broth. Add the salt, thyme, and pepper. Bring to a boil, reduce the heat to maintain a simmer, and cook for about 5 minutes, until thickened.

7. Stir in the milk. Cook for 1 or 2 more minutes, until heated through, and serve.

PER SERVING: Calories: 82; Total fat: 5g; Saturated fat: 1g; Protein: 3g; Carbs: 8g; Sugar: 2g; Fiber: 1g; Cholesterol: 0mg; Sodium: 226mg

Artichoke Dip

SERVES 4 | **PREP TIME:** 10 minutes | **COOK TIME:** 10 minutes

Dips are always in demand when serving crackers, veggies, or pretzels. They add a certain quality to the enjoyment of eating. But some dips may be not as healthy as you think. That's why this artichoke dip, made with low-fat cream cheese and nonfat Greek yogurt, is much healthier than your typical artichoke dip. Better yet, it mixes up in no time for unexpected company or when you simply want a special treat.

1 (8-ounce) package low-fat cream cheese

2 cups plain nonfat Greek yogurt

2 (14-ounce) cans artichoke hearts, drained and coarsely chopped

2 or 3 garlic cloves, minced

1 cup grated Parmesan cheese

½ teaspoon salt

In a medium pot over medium heat, combine the cream cheese, yogurt, artichoke hearts, garlic, Parmesan cheese, and salt. Cook for about 8 minutes, stirring regularly, until the dip starts to bubble, and serve. Refrigerate leftovers in an airtight container for up to 5 days.

PER SERVING: Calories: 262; Total fat: 6g; Saturated fat: 4g; Protein: 25g; Carbs: 27g; Sugar: 16g; Fiber: 5g; Cholesterol: 33mg; Sodium: 432mg

5-Minute Hummus

SERVES 4 | **PREP TIME:** 5 minutes

Made from chickpeas, hummus is a thick Middle Eastern paste or spread used mainly for dipping vegetables or spreading on sandwiches. It's become incredibly popular not only because it's delicious, but also for its versatility and impressive health benefits. This plant-based protein contains a wide variety of vitamins and minerals and is an excellent option for people on a vegetarian or vegan diet. Explore the variations to make your hummus how you like it.

1 (15.5-ounce) can reduced-sodium chickpeas, drained and rinsed

¼ cup tahini

Juice of 2 lemons

2 garlic cloves, minced

1 tablespoon extra-virgin olive oil

½ teaspoon salt

2 to 3 tablespoons water, as needed

1. In a blender or food processor, combine the chickpeas, tahini, lemon juice, garlic, olive oil, and salt. Process until smooth. Stop, scrape down the sides of the blender, and mix again.

2. Add the water and continue to process until the hummus is smooth. Transfer to an airtight container and refrigerate for up to 5 days.

VARIATION TIP: Add about ½ cup sun-dried tomatoes, spinach, or chopped Kalamata olives for a different take on this simple dip.

PER SERVING: Calories: 187; Total fat: 12g; Saturated fat: 2g; Protein: 6g; Carbs: 15g; Sugar: 4g; Fiber: 2g; Cholesterol: 0mg; Sodium: 423mg

Perfect Quinoa Salad

SERVES 6 | **PREP TIME:** 15 minutes | **COOK TIME:** 15 minutes

This quinoa salad is refreshingly crisp and delicious. The blend of cucumber, red bell pepper, red onion, and garlicky olive oil and lemon dressing is similar to tabbouleh, but with gluten-free quinoa instead of bulgur. To remove any bite of bitter oils, rinse the quinoa in a fine-mesh strainer before cooking.

1 cup quinoa, rinsed

1½ cups water

1 cucumber, finely chopped

1 red bell pepper, finely chopped

½ red onion, chopped

½ cup fresh flat-leaf parsley

¼ cup extra-virgin olive oil

Juice of 2 lemons

3 garlic cloves, minced

½ teaspoon salt

¼ teaspoon freshly ground black pepper

1. In a small saucepan over high heat, combine the quinoa and water. Bring to a boil, reduce the heat to low, cover the pot, and cook for 10 to 15 minutes, until the water is absorbed. Turn off the heat, fluff with a fork, re-cover, and let rest for about 5 minutes.

2. Meanwhile, in a large bowl, toss the cucumber, red bell pepper, red onion, and parsley.

3. In a small bowl, whisk the olive oil, lemon juice, garlic, salt, and pepper. Pour the dressing over the vegetables, and toss well to coat. Fold in the quinoa and serve.

VARIATION TIP: Make this a complete meal by adding 1 (15-ounce) can rinsed and drained chickpeas to the salad.

PER SERVING: Calories: 200; Total fat: 10g; Saturated fat: 2g; Protein: 5g; Carbs: 23g; Sugar: 3g; Fiber: 3g; Cholesterol: 0mg; Sodium: 202mg

Simple Brown Rice

SERVES 4 | **PREP TIME:** 5 minutes | **COOK TIME:** 1 hour

Okay, this may be the simplest, most totally hands off, foolproof recipe yet. Just boil, bake, and an hour later you have a truly appetizing and perfect portion of rice—every time. Speaking of portions, high-fiber brown rice does contain carbs, so to control your intake, store it individually in ½-cup serving-size portions. Rice is always a great side when putting together a meal. Add some extra color and flavor with chopped parsley, thinly sliced scallion, or shredded carrot.

1½ cups brown rice

1 teaspoon salt

3 cups boiling water

1. Preheat the oven to 400° F.

2. In a 9-inch baking dish, combine the rice and salt. Pour the boiling water over top. Cover the dish securely with aluminum foil or a lid. Bake for about 1 hour, or until all the water is absorbed.

3. Fluff with a fork and serve.

VARIATION TIP: Brown rice is a simple whole-grain side dish that can round out a meal. Serve it with meat, chicken, and fish dishes along with some steamed vegetables for an easy and filling meal, or mix it with leftover chopped meats and vegetables for a grain bowl. It also goes great with beans for a burrito filling.

PER SERVING: Calories: 258; Total fat: 2g; Saturated fat: 0g; Protein: 5g; Carbs: 54g; Sugar: 0g; Fiber: 2g; Cholesterol: 0mg; Sodium: 584mg

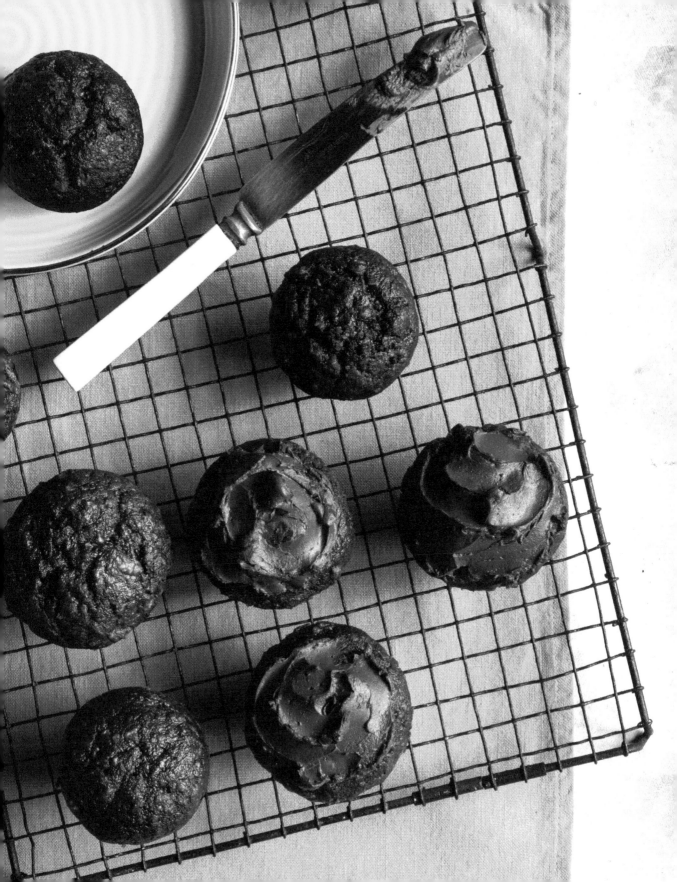

Dessert

Tropical Fruit Salad with Coconut Milk

SERVES 8 | **PREP TIME:** 10 minutes

Here's a perfect side dish to wow and impress your guests. From the pop of colors to the luscious blend of tropical fruit, it's an incredibly easy showstopper, and you can mix and match other fruits such as papaya and strawberries. To save time and energy cutting up fresh pineapple, use precut pineapple or pineapple canned in its own juice. Garnish with toasted flaked or shredded coconut for a crunchy topping, if you like.

2 cups pineapple chunks

2 kiwi fruits, peeled and sliced

1 mango, peeled and chopped

¼ cup canned light coconut milk

1 tablespoon freshly squeezed lime juice

1 tablespoon honey

1. In a medium bowl, toss together the pineapple, kiwi, and mango.

2. In a small bowl, combine the coconut milk, lime juice, and honey, stirring until the honey dissolves. Pour the mixture over the fruits, and toss to coat. Serve immediately or refrigerate in an airtight container for up to 3 days.

PER SERVING: Calories: 70; Total fat: 1g; Saturated fat: 0g; Protein: 1g; Carbs: 17g; Sugar: 14g; Fiber: 2g; Cholesterol: 0mg; Sodium: 2mg

Mango Smoothie

SERVES 2 | **PREP TIME:** 5 minutes

Mango is a favorite fruit of mine, and when blended into a smoothie, it's delicious. This "king of the fruits" is one of the most popular and widely consumed fruits in the world. And it's easy to see why—the golden yellow interior offers a sweet, creamy, unique taste, and when combined with milk and yogurt, it's hard to resist. You can use frozen mango; just thaw for about 15 minutes first. You can even enjoy this smoothie if you follow a vegan diet by substituting almond milk and coconut yogurt for the dairy.

2 cups frozen or fresh chopped mango

½ cup skim milk

½ cup plain nonfat Greek yogurt

In a high-speed blender, combine the mango, milk, and yogurt. Process until smooth, and serve.

VARIATION TIP: If using fresh mango, add a couple of ice cubes to the blender for a thicker smoothie. Also, if you would like a slightly sweeter smoothie, add 1 or 2 teaspoons of honey.

PER SERVING: Calories: 154; Total fat: 1g; Saturated fat: 0g; Protein: 6g; Carbs: 33g; Sugar: 30g; Fiber: 3g; Cholesterol: 2mg; Sodium: 79mg

Spiced Honey Almonds

SERVES 8 | **PREP TIME:** 5 minutes | **COOK TIME:** 15 minutes

These almonds are addictively delicious. The little bit of spice is subtle and surprisingly good. For easy prep and cleanup, be sure to use parchment paper. The cinnamon provides a beneficial boost for blood sugar management. The almonds themselves are a good low-carb, high-fiber, protein-rich food, making them excellent for long-lasting fullness. Make these spiced honey almonds once, and you'll be hooked.

3 tablespoons honey

1 teaspoon ground cinnamon

½ teaspoon ground cayenne pepper

½ teaspoon salt

2 cups almonds

1. Preheat the oven to 325°F. Line a baking sheet with parchment paper. Set aside.

2. In a small saucepan over medium heat, warm the honey until softened.

3. Add the cinnamon, cayenne, and salt, and stir well to combine.

4. Add the almonds, and stir until coated. Spread the almonds on the prepared baking sheet in a single layer, and bake for 15 minutes.

5. Remove and let cool on the baking sheet, then serve or transfer to a serving bowl or airtight container. Store at room temperature.

PER SERVING: Calories: 162; Total fat: 12g; Saturated fat: 1g; Protein: 5g; Carbs: 12g; Sugar: 8g; Fiber: 3g; Cholesterol: 0mg; Sodium: 148mg

Chocolate Pudding

SERVES 2 | **PREP TIME:** 5 minutes, plus 1 hour to chill | **COOK TIME:** 15 minutes

Chocolate Pudding—always a welcomed treat! This dairy-free alternative using almond milk will also be a delight, as everyone will ooh and ahh over its smooth, rich taste. Company will think you worked for hours perfecting it, but you'll know all it took was mere minutes. To help with the thickening, refrigerate to chill once it's been cooked.

1 cup almond milk

2 tablespoons honey

2 tablespoons unsweetened cocoa powder

2 tablespoons cornstarch

1 teaspoon vanilla extract

Pinch salt

In a saucepan over medium-high heat, stir together the almond milk, honey, cocoa powder, cornstarch, vanilla, and salt. Bring to a boil, reduce the heat to maintain a simmer, and cook for about 10 minutes, or until thickened. Transfer to a bowl, cover with plastic wrap, and chill for at least 1 hour before serving.

PER SERVING: Calories: 155; Total fat: 4g; Saturated fat: 0g; Protein: 2g; Carbs: 29g; Sugar: 3g; Fiber: 18g; Cholesterol: 0mg; Sodium: 260mg

Blueberries with Sweet Cashew Cream

SERVES 4 | **PREP TIME:** 10 minutes, plus 30 minutes to soak

This dessert is healthy—but no one would ever guess. It's a great dessert for summer, as it requires no cooking and is super-easy to make. It's a great last-minute addition to a party spread when you need something a little lighter on the dessert table.

1 cup raw cashews

2 tablespoons maple syrup

¼ to ½ cup unsweetened vanilla almond milk

2 tablespoons freshly squeezed lemon juice

½ teaspoon vanilla extract

Pinch salt

1 pint fresh blueberries

1. In a small bowl, combine the cashews with enough hot water to cover. Soak for 30 minutes.

2. Drain the cashews, and transfer to a food processor. Add the maple syrup, ¼ cup of almond milk, and the lemon juice, vanilla, and salt. Process until smooth, adding more almond milk as needed.

3. Serve the cashew cream with the blueberries. Refrigerate any unused cashew cream separately in an airtight container for 3 to 4 days.

VARIATION TIP: This works great with blueberries, as well as other berries, because they hold their shape well. Try blackberries, strawberries, or raspberries for a change.

PER SERVING: Calories: 265; Total fat: 14g; Saturated fat: 2g; Protein: 6g; Carbs: 30g; Sugar: 16g; Fiber: 4g; Cholesterol: 0mg; Sodium: 56mg

Chocolate-Dipped Strawberries

SERVES 6 | **PREP TIME:** 15 minutes, plus 30 minutes to rest | **COOK TIME:** About 1 minute

Nothing satisfies a sweet tooth quite like strawberries dipped in chocolate. This very simple recipe is perfect for increasing fruit consumption, and it's guaranteed that everyone will want to do their share of dipping. Dark baking chocolate contains up to 2 to 3 times more flavanol-rich cocoa solids, good for relaxing blood vessels and improving blood flow, which can help lower blood pressure.

1 pint fresh strawberries, rinsed individually and thoroughly dried with a towel

1½ ounces dark baking chocolate, chopped into small pieces

1. Line a baking sheet with parchment paper. Set aside.

2. Set the dried strawberries on a clean, dry towel to continue to air dry while you prepare the chocolate.

3. Place the chocolate in a microwave-safe jar or bowl, and microwave on medium power for 30 seconds. Stir the chocolate and continue to microwave at medium power in 20-second intervals, stirring after each, until melted.

4. Holding the top of each strawberry, dip the berries into the chocolate and place on the prepared baking sheet. Let rest at room temperature until hardened, or refrigerate for 30 minutes. Serve immediately or refrigerate in an airtight container for up to 3 days.

VARIATION TIP: Chocolate tastes great with a variety of fruits, such as pineapple, melons, and bananas, so feel free to try them all.

PER SERVING: Calories: 54; Total fat: 2g; Saturated fat: 1g; Protein: 1g; Carbs: 9g; Sugar: 6g; Fiber: 1g; Cholesterol: 0mg; Sodium: 3mg

Dark Chocolate Drops

MAKES 24 PIECES | **PREP TIME:** 10 minutes, plus 30 minutes to rest | **COOK TIME:** About 1 minute

Combine heart-healthy dark chocolate with a sprinkling of dried fruit, chopped nuts, and seeds, and you've got a super simple way to please your sweet tooth. These made-to-order drops (customize them to your tastes) are a fun way to create a tasty snack-like dessert you can eat without feeling guilty. Keep portion sizes small, and use these as an occasional treat.

8 ounces dark chocolate, chopped

3 tablespoons dried fruit, such as cranberries, blueberries, cherries, pineapple, or mango

3 tablespoons chopped nuts, such as almonds, walnuts, hazelnuts, pistachios, or peanuts

1 tablespoon seeds, such as sunflower, chia, hemp, or flaxseed

1. Line a baking sheet with parchment paper. Set aside.

2. Place the chocolate in a microwave-safe bowl, and microwave on medium power for 30 seconds. Stir and continue to microwave in 20-second intervals, stirring after each, until melted. Drop teaspoon-size spoonfuls of chocolate onto the prepared baking sheet, making rounds that spread to about 2 inches in diameter.

3. Sprinkle the fruit, nuts, and seeds over the chocolate. Let sit at room temperature until it hardens, or refrigerate for 30 minutes. Serve immediately or transfer to an airtight container and refrigerate for up to 2 weeks.

PER SERVING (2 DROPS): Calories: 111; Total fat: 7g; Saturated fat: 3g; Protein: 1g; Carbs: 14g; Sugar: 11g; Fiber: 0g; Cholesterol: 0mg; Sodium: 7mg

Easy Berry Sorbet

SERVES 6 | **PREP TIME:** 10 minutes, plus 2 hours to freeze | **COOK TIME:** 5 minutes

Berries are one of the very best fruits to eat. Loaded with antioxidants and high in fiber, berries may help improve blood sugar and, best of all, are very tasty. While fresh berries are always good, sometimes it's nice to try them prepared differently, such as in a sorbet. This homemade frozen treat using real fruit (fresh or frozen) is simply perfect. Colorful, satisfying, and healthy, it may replace your store-bought sorbets forever. You control the amount of sugar—follow the recipe or reduce the sugar to just 2 tablespoons. Just be sure to also reduce the water to 2 tablespoons.

¼ cup sugar

1 thyme sprig

¼ cup water

1 pound fresh or frozen raspberries

8 ounces fresh or frozen blueberries

1. Line a rimmed baking sheet with parchment paper or wax paper. Set aside.

2. In a small saucepan over medium heat, combine the sugar, thyme, and water. Heat, stirring, until the sugar dissolves. Remove from the heat, and let the simple syrup cool. Once cool, remove the thyme sprig.

3. In a high-speed blender, combine the raspberries, blueberries, and simple syrup. Process until smooth. Pour the mixture through a fine-mesh strainer or cheesecloth set over a bowl to remove the seeds. Transfer the purée to the prepared baking sheet, and freeze for 2 to 3 hours, or until solid.

4. Break the sorbet into pieces, place them in a blender, and process again to your desired texture. Serve immediately, or freeze again until ready to use.

TECHNIQUE TIP: As the fruit freezes, ice crystals develop. Blending the sorbet twice will make it smooth and creamy.

PER SERVING: Calories: 131; Total fat: 0g; Saturated fat: 0g; Protein: 1g; Carbs: 34g; Sugar: 29g; Fiber: 4g; Cholesterol: 0mg; Sodium: 1mg

Stuffed Dates

MAKES 24 DATES | **PREP TIME:** 15 minutes

When your sweet cravings strike, consider curbing them with a fun snack made of dates. Dates are a high-fiber dried fruit and a good source of potassium and copper. If prepped on a weekend, these will last the entire week when refrigerated. To save time, consider buying pitted dates.

24 Medjool dates

4 ounces low-fat cream cheese, at room temperature

¼ teaspoon ground nutmeg

¼ teaspoon dried ginger

24 raw almonds

1. Using a paring knife, slice each date lengthwise just enough to remove its pit. Set the dates aside.

2. In a small bowl, stir together the cream cheese, nutmeg, and ginger until well combined. Stuff each date with about 1 teaspoon of the cream cheese mixture, and top each with 1 almond.

3. Chill until ready to serve. Refrigerate in an airtight container for up to 1 week.

PER SERVING (2 STUFFED DATES): Calories: 211; Total fat: 5g; Saturated fat: 2g; Protein: 2g; Carbs: 43g; Sugar: 34g; Fiber: 4g; Cholesterol: 10mg; Sodium: 40mg

Carrot Cake

SERVES 12 | **PREP TIME:** 10 minutes | **COOK TIME:** 25 minutes

A good Carrot Cake is hard to beat—and this one doesn't disappoint. Much lower in sugar than traditional Carrot Cake, this lighter version is made mostly with whole-wheat flour, but with just enough sweetness to satisfy. If desired, top with the frosting from the Sweet Potato Cake (page 135). Keep the portion size small, and you can still enjoy this delightful treat.

Nonstick cooking spray

1½ cups whole-wheat pastry flour

½ cup all-purpose flour

1½ cups grated carrot

½ cup sugar

2 teaspoons baking powder

1 teaspoon baking soda

½ teaspoon salt

4 large eggs, lightly beaten

¼ cup canola oil

1. Preheat the oven to 350°F. Spray a 9-inch baking pan with cooking spray. Set aside.

2. In a medium bowl, stir together the whole-wheat pastry and all-purpose flours, carrot, sugar, baking powder, baking soda, and salt.

3. Add the eggs and canola oil, and stir until the flour is completely mixed in. Transfer the thick batter to the prepared pan. Bake for 20 to 25 minutes, until browned and a toothpick inserted into the center comes out clean.

4. Slice into 12 pieces and serve, or store loosely covered at room temperature for 1 to 2 days, refrigerate covered for up to 1 week, or wrap in aluminum foil and place in a freezer bag and freeze for up to 3 months.

PER SERVING: Calories: 173; Total fat: 7g; Saturated fat: 1g; Protein: 4g; Carbs: 25g; Sugar: 9g; Fiber: 2g; Cholesterol: 62mg; Sodium: 235mg

Almond Power Balls

SERVES 6 | **PREP TIME:** 10 minutes, plus 1 hour to chill

These Almond Power Balls are a powerhouse of nutritional goodness. Loaded with energizing protein and healthy fat, this treat will get you up and moving. With just enough natural sweetness to satisfy, these are great to take along when out and about to keep hunger at bay. If your dates are dry, soak them in hot water for 15 minutes before making the recipe and they'll soften up perfectly.

1½ cups raw almonds

½ cup tightly packed pitted Medjool dates

2 tablespoons almond or peanut butter

Pinch sea salt

¼ cup unsweetened shredded coconut

1. In a high-speed blender or food processor, pulse the almonds until they are coarse crumbs. Add the dates, and process until finely chopped.

2. Add the almond butter and salt, and process until mixed. While processing, add water, 1 teaspoon at a time, until the dough comes together. Roll the dough into 1½-inch balls.

3. Place the coconut in a small bowl, and roll the balls in it, pressing to coat. Refrigerate for about 1 hour before serving. Refrigerate in an airtight container for up to 2 weeks.

PER SERVING (2 BALLS): Calories: 269; Total fat: 20g; Saturated fat: 6g; Protein: 8g; Carbs: 19g; Sugar: 11g; Fiber: 6g; Cholesterol: 0mg; Sodium: 67mg

Roasted Spiced Pears

SERVES 4 | **PREP TIME:** 5 minutes | **COOK TIME:** 30 minutes

A good pear is one of the best fruits around. When baked with a little cinnamon (good for blood glucose control), honey, and protein-rich pistachios, these will have you set for excellent eating. Pears are a great source of fiber and vitamin C, with only 100 calories and zero fat. Choose Bosc or Anjou pears—best for baking—and, if desired, serve with ice cream or vanilla Greek yogurt.

2 pears, halved

¼ teaspoon ground cinnamon

1 tablespoon honey

¼ cup crushed pistachios

1. Preheat the oven to 350°F.

2. Using a spoon, scoop out and discard the pears' seeds. Sprinkle the pear halves with cinnamon, drizzle on the honey, and sprinkle the pistachios over the top. Place the pears on a baking sheet, and bake for 30 minutes, until tender. Let cool and serve.

PER SERVING: Calories: 136; Total fat: 5g; Saturated fat: 1g; Protein: 2g; Carbs: 23g; Sugar: 15g; Fiber: 4g; Cholesterol: 0mg; Sodium: 2mg

Apple Crisp

SERVES 6 | **PREP TIME:** 15 minutes | **COOK TIME:** 45 minutes

Low in sugar but with lots of taste, this Apple Crisp is a great way to serve apples. Fortunately, there are lots of apples to choose from that work best when baked—Cortland, Rome, Braeburn, Honeycrisp, and Fuji, to name a few. Once the apples are peeled, put the ingredients together quickly to prevent browning. Consider adding chopped pecans or walnuts to the topping to provide a nice crunchy finish.

FOR THE APPLE FILLING

Nonstick cooking spray

5 medium apples, peeled, cored, and sliced

2 tablespoons freshly squeezed lemon juice

2 tablespoons sugar

½ teaspoon ground cinnamon

1 tablespoon whole-wheat flour

1 tablespoon butter, melted

Pinch salt

FOR THE CRISP TOPPING

1 cup quick-cooking oats

¼ cup whole-wheat flour

¼ cup sugar

½ teaspoon ground cinnamon

¼ teaspoon salt

4 tablespoons butter, cut into ¼-inch pieces

TO MAKE THE APPLE FILLING

1. Preheat the oven to 350° F. Spray an 8-inch baking dish with cooking spray. Set aside.

2. In a large bowl, toss together the apples, lemon juice, sugar, cinnamon, flour, butter, and salt. Transfer the mixture to the prepared dish.

TO MAKE THE CRISP TOPPING

1. In a small bowl, combine the oats, flour, sugar, cinnamon, salt, and butter. Using a pastry blender or two forks, cut the butter into smaller pieces and mix well.

2. Using your hands, crumble the topping over the apples. Bake for 45 minutes, until the top is browned and the apples are tender.

3. Slice into 6 pieces and serve, or store loosely covered at room temperature for 3 days or up to 1 week in the refrigerator.

PER SERVING: Calories: 287; Total fat: 11g; Saturated fat: 6g; Protein: 3g; Carbs: 48g; Sugar: 32g; Fiber: 6g; Cholesterol: 25mg; Sodium: 169mg

Sweet Potato Cake

SERVES 10 | **PREP TIME:** 15 minutes | **COOK TIME:** 30 minutes

Never had Sweet Potato Cake? You're in for a treat. Reminiscent of Carrot Cake (page 131), this luscious dessert brings a less intense sweetness to the table, but still plenty of flavor. Thanks to the sweet potato living up to its name, only ¼ cup of sugar is needed rather than the more typical 2 cups in other cake recipes. When choosing just the right sweet potatoes, go with bright orange–fleshed varieties. All that orange means beta-carotene, a potent antioxidant.

FOR THE CAKE

Nonstick cooking spray

2 small sweet potatoes, peeled and shredded

1 cup whole-wheat flour

1 cup all-purpose flour

¼ cup sugar

2 teaspoons baking powder

2 teaspoons ground cinnamon

½ teaspoon ground ginger

½ teaspoon salt

1 cup unsweetened applesauce

¼ cup canola oil

2 large eggs

FOR THE FROSTING

1 (8-ounce) package low-fat cream cheese, at room temperature

¼ cup honey

1 teaspoon vanilla extract

TO MAKE THE CAKE

1. Preheat the oven to 350° F. Spray a 9-inch baking dish with cooking spray. Set aside.

2. In a large bowl, stir together the sweet potatoes, whole-wheat and all-purpose flours, sugar, baking powder, cinnamon, ginger, and salt.

3. In a medium bowl, whisk the applesauce, oil, and eggs. Pour the wet mixture into the dry mixture, and stir until combined. Transfer the mixture to the prepared baking dish. Bake for 25 to 30 minutes, until the top is browned and a toothpick inserted into the middle comes out clean.

4. Let cool completely before frosting.

TO MAKE THE FROSTING

In a small bowl, combine the cream cheese, honey, and vanilla. Using a handheld electric mixer, beat well until smooth and combined. Frost the cake. Slice into 10 pieces and serve, or loosely cover the completed cake and refrigerate for up to 1 week.

PER SERVING: Calories: 306; Total fat: 15g; Saturated fat: 6g; Protein: 6g; Carbs: 39g; Sugar: 16g; Fiber: 3g; Cholesterol: 62mg; Sodium: 214mg

Chocolate-Zucchini Cupcakes

MAKES 12 CUPCAKES | **PREP TIME:** 15 minutes | **COOK TIME:** 25 minutes

For whatever reason, chocolate and zucchini go well together, sort of like apples and peanut butter or macaroni and cheese. This is a great recipe for whipping up quick and easy. Use only one bowl for mixing, and no need to peel the zucchini—leave it on for extra fiber and nutrients. This makes a fun dessert for friends or family, or whenever you'd like a sweet treat.

FOR THE CUPCAKES

Nonstick cooking spray

2 cups shredded zucchini

1 cup whole-wheat flour

1 cup all-purpose flour

2 large eggs

¾ cup granulated sugar

½ cup unsweetened applesauce

½ cup unsweetened cocoa powder

¼ cup canola oil

1 teaspoon baking powder

½ teaspoon salt

FOR THE FROSTING

8 ounces low-fat cream cheese, at room temperature

2 tablespoons butter, at room temperature

½ cup unsweetened cocoa powder

1 cup powdered sugar

1 teaspoon vanilla extract

TO MAKE THE CUPCAKES

1. Preheat the oven to 325° F. Spray a muffin tin with cooking spray. Set aside.

2. In a large bowl, combine the zucchini, whole-wheat and all-purpose flours, eggs, granulated sugar, applesauce, cocoa powder, oil, baking powder, and salt. Mix well. Fill the muffin cups with the batter, and bake for 25 minutes, until a toothpick inserted into the center of one comes out clean.

3. Remove from the oven, and let cool before frosting.

TO MAKE THE FROSTING

In a bowl or stand mixer, beat the cream cheese and butter until well combined. Stir in the cocoa powder, powdered sugar, and vanilla extract. Frost the cooled cupcakes and serve, or refrigerate the finished cupcakes in an airtight container for up to 1 week.

INGREDIENT TIP: If you have a high-speed blender, you can make powdered sugar at home. For 1 cup powdered sugar, start with about ½ cup granulated sugar and process until it resembles a fine, fluffy powder.

PER SERVING: Calories: 319; Total fat: 15g; Saturated fat: 7g; Protein: 7g; Carbs: 44g; Sugar: 24g; Fiber: 4g; Cholesterol: 57mg; Sodium: 182mg

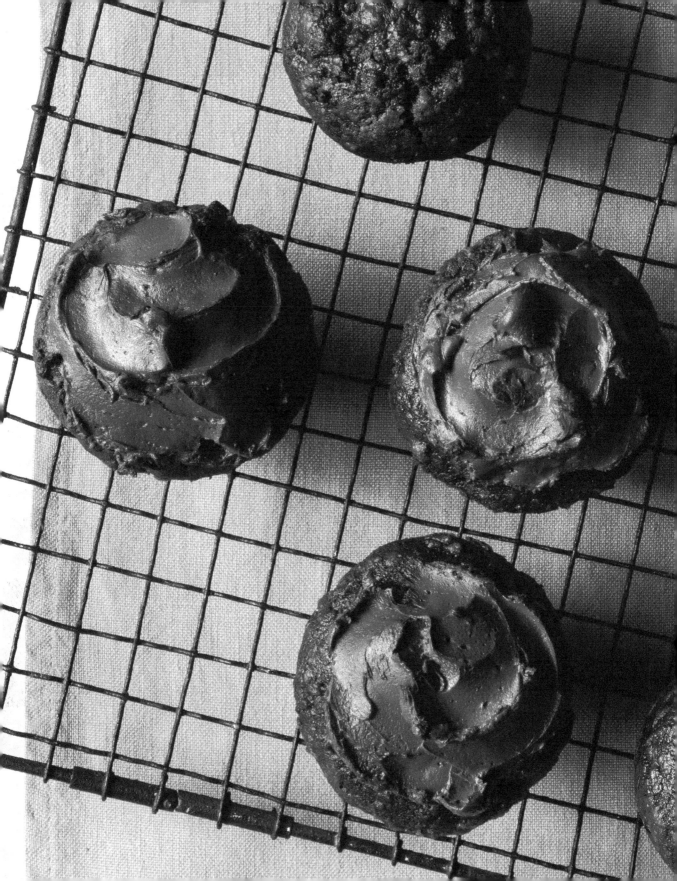

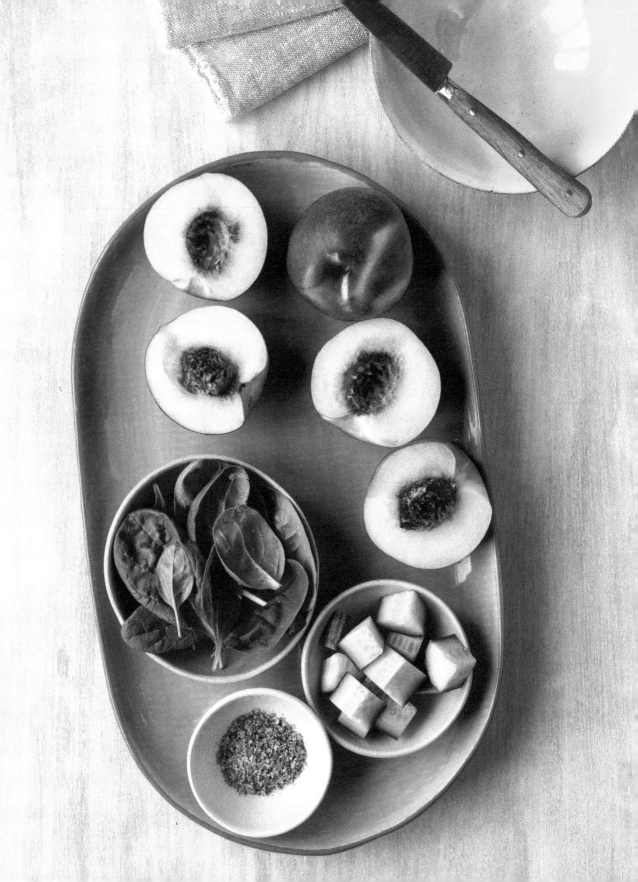

Measurement Conversions

VOLUME EQUIVALENTS (LIQUID)

US STANDARD	US STANDARD (OUNCES)	METRIC (APPROXIMATE)
2 tablespoons	1 fl. oz.	30 mL
¼ cup	2 fl. oz.	60 mL
½ cup	4 fl. oz.	120 mL
1 cup	8 fl. oz.	240 mL
1½ cups	12 fl. oz.	355 mL
2 cups or 1 pint	16 fl. oz.	475 mL
4 cups or 1 quart	32 fl. oz.	1 L
1 gallon	128 fl. oz.	4 L

OVEN TEMPERATURES

FAHRENHEIT (F)	CELSIUS (C) (APPROXIMATE)
250° F	120° C
300° F	150° C
325° F	165° C
350° F	180° C
375° F	190° C
400° F	200° C
425° F	220° C
450° F	230° C

VOLUME EQUIVALENTS (DRY)

US STANDARD	METRIC (APPROXIMATE)
⅛ teaspoon	0.5 mL
¼ teaspoon	1 mL
½ teaspoon	2 mL
¾ teaspoon	4 mL
1 teaspoon	5 mL
1 tablespoon	15 mL
¼ cup	59 mL
⅓ cup	79 mL
½ cup	118 mL
⅔ cup	156 mL
¾ cup	177 mL
1 cup	235 mL
2 cups or 1 pint	475 mL
3 cups	700 mL
4 cups or 1 quart	1 L

WEIGHT EQUIVALENTS

US STANDARD	METRIC (APPROXIMATE)
½ ounce	15 g
1 ounce	30 g
2 ounces	60 g
4 ounces	115 g
8 ounces	225 g
12 ounces	340 g
16 ounces or 1 pound	455 g

The Dirty Dozen
and the Clean Fifteen™

A nonprofit environmental watchdog organization called Environmental Working Group (EWG) looks at data supplied by the US Department of Agriculture (USDA) and the Food and Drug Administration (FDA) about pesticide residues. Each year it compiles a list of the best and worst pesticide loads found in commercial crops. You can use these lists to decide which fruits and vegetables to buy organic to minimize your exposure to pesticides and which produce is considered safe enough to buy conventionally. This does not mean they are pesticide-free, though, so wash these fruits and vegetables thoroughly. The list is updated annually, and you can find it online at EWG.org/FoodNews.

DIRTY DOZEN™

1. strawberries
2. spinach
3. kale
4. nectarines
5. apples
6. grapes
7. peaches
8. cherries
9. pears
10. tomatoes
11. celery
12. potatoes

†Additionally, nearly three-quarters of hot pepper samples contained pesticide residues.

CLEAN FIFTEEN™

1. avocados
2. sweet corn*
3. pineapples
4. sweet peas (frozen)
5. onions
6. papayas*
7. eggplants
8. asparagus
9. kiwis
10. cabbages
11. cauliflower
12. cantaloupes
13. broccoli
14. mushrooms
15. honeydew melons

* A small amount of sweet corn, papaya, and summer squash sold in the United States is produced from genetically modified seeds. Buy organic varieties of these crops if you want to avoid genetically modified produce.

Resources

Here are a few resources to help you and your loved ones learn more about prediabetes.

Academy of Nutrition and Dietetics (EatRight.org): A national organization for registered dietitians in the United States that is the most credible source of nutrition information.

American Diabetes Association (Diabetes.org): A nonprofit organization that seeks to educate the public about both prediabetes and diabetes and help those affected by it by funding research to manage, cure, and prevent diabetes.

American Heart Association (Heart.org): A national organization in the United States that funds cardiovascular medical research, educates consumers on healthy living regarding diet, exercise, and stress management, and promotes cardiac care.

Centers for Disease Control and Prevention (CDC.gov/diabetes): A US federal agency that conducts and supports health promotion and prevention with the goal of improving public health.

National Diabetes Education Program (NDEP.NIH.gov): Started by the National Institutes of Health and Centers for Disease Control in 1997, this program educates the public about the risks of diabetes with the goal to reduce the illness and deaths caused by it and its complications.

National Diabetes Information Clearinghouse (Diabetes.NIDDK.NIH.gov): An information dissemination service of the National Institute of Diabetes and Digestive and Kidney Diseases (NIDDK). The clearinghouse responds to inquiries about diabetes, provides referrals to health professionals, and offers publications.

Stop Diabetes (StopDiabetes.com): A movement working to end the devastating toll that diabetes takes on the lives of millions of individuals and families.

United States Department of Agriculture's MyPlate (ChooseMyPlate.gov): MyPlate helps illustrate the five food groups of a healthy diet using the familiar image of a place setting. The website provides information on eating on a budget, MyPlate tip sheets, quizzes, and recipes.

References

American Diabetes Association. "American Diabetes Association Issues New Recommendations on Physical Activity and Exercise for People with Diabetes." October 25, 2016. Accessed December 29, 2018. www.diabetes.org/newsroom/press-releases/2016/ada-issues-new-recommendations-on-physical-activity-and-exercise.html.

American Diabetes Association. "Diagnosing Diabetes and Learning About Prediabetes." Accessed December 31, 2018. http://diabetes.org/diabetes-basics/diagnosis/.

American Diabetes Association. "Fitness." Accessed December 30, 2018. http://www.diabetes.org/food-and-fitness/fitness/.

Centers for Disease Control and Prevention. "More Than 100 million Americans Have Diabetes or Prediabetes." July 18, 2017. Accessed December 21, 2018. www.cdc.gov/media/releases/2017/p0718-diabetes-report.html.

Centers for Disease Control and Prevention. "National Diabetes Statistics Report." February 24, 2018. Accessed December 20, 2018. www.cdc.gov/diabetes/data/statistics/statistics-report.html.

Gardner, B. "Making Health Habitual: The Psychology of 'Habit-Formation' and General Practice." *British Journal of General Practice* 62, no. 605 (December 2012): 664–666. Accessed December 28, 2018. doi:10.3399/bjgp12X659466.

Knowler, W. C., S. E. Fowler, R. D. Hamman, C. A. Christophi, H. J. Hoffman, A. T. Brenneman, J. O. Brown-Friday, et al. "10-Year Follow-Up of Diabetes Incidence and Weight Loss in the Diabetes Prevention Program Outcomes Study." *The Lancet* 374, no. 9702 (November 2009): 1677–86. Accessed December 20, 2018. doi:10.1016/S0140-6736(09)61457-4.

Lean, M. E., W. S. Leslie, A. C. Barnes, N. Brosnahan, G. Thom, and L. McCombie. "Primary Care-Led Weight Management for Remission of Type 2 Diabetes (DiRECT): An Open-Label, Cluster-Randomised Trial." *The Lancet* 391, no. 10120 (February 2018): 541–551. Accessed December 21, 2018. doi:https://doi.org/10.1016/S0140-6736(17)33102-1.

National Institute of Alcohol Abuse and Alcoholism. "Are Women More Vulnerable to Alcohol's Effects?" no. 46 (December 1999). Accessed December 21, 2018. https://pubs.niaaa.nih.gov/publications/aa46.htm.

National Institute of Alcohol Abuse and Alcoholism. "Women and Alcohol." Accessed December 28, 2018. https://pubs.niaaa.nih.gov/publications /womensfact/womensfact.htm.

National Sleep Foundation. "Healthy Sleep Tips." Accessed December 30, 2018. https://www.sleepfoundation.org/sleep-tools-tips/healthy-sleep-tips.

Office of Disease Prevention and Health Promotion. *2015–2020 Dietary Guidelines for Americans*, 8th edition. "Appendix 2. Estimated Calorie Needs per Day, by Age, Sex, and Physical Activity Level." Accessed December 21, 2018. https://health.gov /dietaryguidelines/2015/guidelines/appendix-2/.

Office of Disease Prevention and Health Promotion. *2015–2020 Dietary Guidelines for Americans*, 8th edition. "Key Recommendations: Components of Healthy Eating Patterns." Accessed December 21, 2018. https://health.gov/dietaryguidelines/2015 /guidelines/chapter-1/key-recommendations/.

Sharecare and Gallup. *2017 State and Community Rankings for the Prevalence of Diabetes—Gallup Sharecare Well-Being Index*. "Sharecare and Gallup Announce 2017 State and Community Rankings for Diabetes Prevalence." November 13, 2018. Accessed December 20, 2018. https://about.sharecare.com/press-releases /sharecare-and-gallup-announce-2017-state-and-community-rankings-for -diabetes-prevalence.

The Sleep Advisor. "Is It Really Better to Sleep in a Cold Room?" Accessed January 25, 2019. https://www.sleepadvisor.org/sleeping-in-a-cold-room/.

Tuso, P. "Prediabetes and Lifestyle Modifications: Time to Prevent a Preventable Disease." *The Permanente Journal* 18, no. 3 (Summer 2014): 88–93. Accessed December 20, 2018. doi:10.7812/TPP/14-002.

Index

Acknowledgments

I AM FILLED WITH DEEP GRATITUDE and appreciation for the opportunities that have come my way in my career as a registered dietitian. To be able to write a book for those with prediabetes, helping them on their journey to good health, is a privilege I cherish.

There are many people I want to thank for making this book possible. First, a huge thank you goes to my editors, Vanessa Putt and Bridget Fitzgerald from Callisto Media, for their patient and encouraging guidance on bringing this book to life. Other special thanks go to my creative and talented recipe developer, Katherine Green. Working with each of you was an absolute pleasure and made this entire process effortless.

Lastly, to my loving, supportive, and patient husband, Casey, who puts up with my tremendous workload, graciously allowing me to pursue my dreams.

About the Author

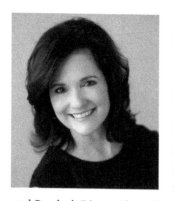

CHERYL MUSSATTO, MS, RD, LD, is a Kansas-based registered dietitian who holds a bachelor's degree in dietetics and institutional management from Kansas State University and a master's degree in dietetics and nutrition from the University of Kansas. Cheryl works at an endocrinology clinic where she has counseled more than 1,000 patients and is an adjunct professor at a community college and a freelance writer. Her work has appeared in various media outlets including *U.S. News and World Report* and *Reader's Digest*. Cheryl is also the blogger behind *Eat Well to Be Well*, where she inspires, teaches, and keeps her followers up to date on the latest developments in nutrition. She is the author of *The Nourished Brain: The Latest Science on Food's Power for Protecting the Brain from Alzheimer's and Dementia*. Cheryl lives in northeast Kansas with her husband, two dogs, and four pygmy goats. Learn more at EatWellToBeWellRD.com.

CPSIA information can be obtained
at www.ICGtesting.com
Printed in the USA
BVHW050359220519
548919BV00002B/2